Body Toning for Women

The contents of this book were carefully researched. However, all information is supplied without liability. Neither the author nor the publisher will be liable for possible disadvantages or damages resulting from this book.

BODY TONING
FOR WOMEN

Meyer & Meyer Sport

British Library Cataloguing in Publication Data
A catalogue record for this book is available from the British Library.

Body Toning for Women
Maidenhead: Meyer & Meyer Sport (UK) Ltd., 2016
ISBN: 978-1-78255-071-6

© 2015 by Meyer & Meyer Sport (UK) Ltd.
Aachen, Auckland, Beirut, Cairo, Cape Town, Dubai, Hägendorf, Hong Kong,
Indianapolis, Manila, New Delhi, Singapore, Sydney, Tehran, Vienna
Member of the World Sport Publishers' Association (WSPA)
Manufacturing: Print Consult GmbH, Munich, Germany
ISBN: 978-1-78255-071-6
E-Mail: info@m-m-sports.com
www.m-m-sports.com

TABLE OF CONTENTS

YOU ARE **YOUR** OWN **GYM**

This book will help you create your dream body; the exercises will tone you and sculpt you in all the right areas to create the body you want.

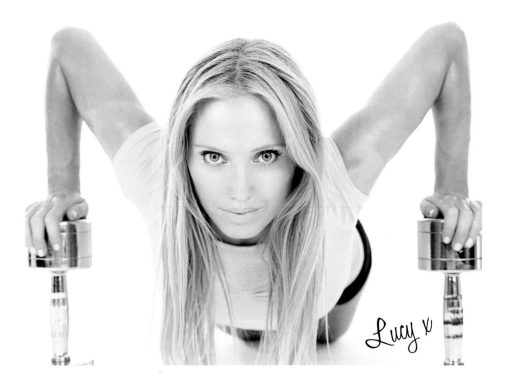

INTRODUCTION

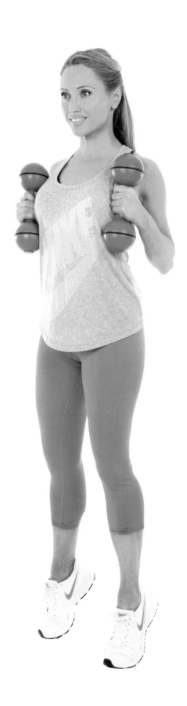

WHAT YOU WILL LOVE ABOUT THIS BOOK

○ EVERY MOVE WILL ALSO HELP YOU BURN FAT, as these specially designed women's toning exercises of mine help activate more muscle tissues, meaning your body will be always burning a higher rate of calories.

○ EVERY MOVE CAN BE DONE ABSOLUTELY ANYWHERE, so if you are away for a girly weekend, are on a business trip or live in a tiny studio apartment, don't worry as you can do every move in my book in the smallest space. This book is your portable gym.

○ IT GIVES YOU TIME BACK. So many minutes are lost driving to gym, attending classes that are way too long or committing to set timetables. In this book I teach you how less is actually more, and you can get super amazing results in a short time, giving you more time back to just enjoy life.

○ GOT IT and by this I mean you will totally understand each exercise and have 100 per cent confidence that you know what you are doing is working. So many other programmes are too complicated, and even the gym can be intimidating because you feel as if you are on stage, performing for all other members, and so can easily perform an exercise wrong. With this book, you will totally get all the exercises and feel 100 per cent confident you are doing them correctly.

○ SAVES YOU MONEY because with this book, all you will ever need is you! There is no need to invest a single penny, so there is no need for expensive gym memberships, fitness classes or expensive, gimmick fitness gadgets.

○ BEST OF ALL, IT GIVES RESULTS. Stick to what I recommend, and I can say, hand on heart, you will feel incredible, will look amazing and will become hooked on living a healthy lifestyle.

Part 1

1   ABOUT TONING

With over 20 years' experience in the fitness industry I keep getting asked the same question: How do I tone up? This is why I decided to write a book showing women how they can tone up and get their dream body. This book contains toning moves that will help to sculpt and create a feminine shape in as little as 21 days. It will give you the confidence to know exactly how to perform each move. The 10 exercises created for each body part—butt, thighs, abs, bust, back and arms—will allow you to create and sculpt your perfect body.

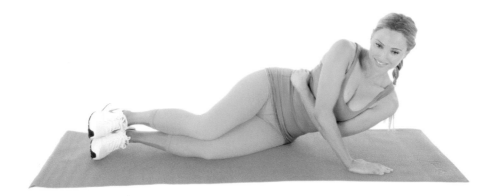

We are unique in the blueprint of our body shape, and not one of us is the same. What is one woman's bugbear, such as the arms, may be another woman's favourite asset. This book allows you to tailor your workout to tone and tighten your body in all the particular areas you want, and it provides you with a vast selection of toning exercises so that you can continually update your routines and never get bored. And this will also allow for quicker results.

HOW YOUR MUSCLES WORK

Let's first look at understanding what toning, also known as strength training, is. As I always say to my clients, **knowledge is power**, so instead of just showing you the exercises, I want to explain how your body reacts to these moves and why we get the results we do.

Toning is also known as strength or resistance training. All of these mean the same thing—a movement in which you use an external force (weights or your own body weight) on a muscle or group of muscles in a range of movement, repeating this range of movement to allow the muscle to grow and become stronger. This is what sculpts and shapes your muscles and also increases the calories your muscles burn.

The reason why toning exercises are a great way to help with fat loss is that the more toned your muscles are, the more calories your body burns. A good way to visualise this is to think of toned muscles as being hyperactive and full of energy, burning lots of calories, whereas untoned muscles would be very inactive and sedentary, burning very few calories.

So every time you do my exercises presented in this book, not only are you sculpting that specific body part, but you are also increasing the amount of calories that muscle will burn off, so it is a win—win situation.

TONING TO KEEP A FEMININE SHAPE

Many women shy away from bodyweight training (which is another name for toning) for fear that they might build up big, bulky muscles, but this is far from being the case, and indeed it would be very hard to achieve, as women don't have the same level of testosterone that men have which enables men to build muscle bulk. To achieve muscle bulk you would require a very specific intense workout and would have to lift extremely heavy weights for a certain amount of reps, and this training would be combined with a specific diet. You would have to put in many hours and a lot of effort to achieve that effect, so you can be safely assured you will not bulk up from the exercises in this book. This book is about creating a sexy, feminine, sculpted body in just 21 days.

FREQUENTLY ASKED QUESTIONS: STRENGTH TRAINING

Question: Will strength training help me to lose weight?

Answer: 100 percent YES. After the age of 30, and in some cases late 20s, our body's ability to burn calories starts to slow down if we are inactive, because our body assumes we don't really use our muscles, and so it slowly starts to reduce the energy they put out. Hence many women in their 30s start to find the weight creeping on, even if they are eating less. Yet adding strength and bodyweight toning workouts engage the muscles, and they become more metabolically active, which means they burn more calories. And the more frequently you do this, the more they stay at this rate. Eventually they get the message and stay fully charged on an ongoing basis (meaning you are burning calories at a faster rate, just like you did in your 20s). So this is a fine example of how exercise really can turn back the body clock.

Question: Is there any exercise I can do to help prevent osteoporosis?

Answer: Yes. Every time you perform a toning exercise you help not only to sculpt your way to a sexy body, but you also build stronger and denser bones. As we age our bones have an increasing risk of suffering from osteoporosis, which is when the bones become brittle and are more likely to fracture and break. When we exercise and use some form of resistance against the body, we create a chemical reaction within the minerals of the bones, and this stimulates the bones to become stronger. So this is another reason to do these exercises, because they will help keep your bones strong.

Question: Can strength training help with poor posture?

Answer: Yes. Posture is something that can instantly add 10 years to you or take 10 years off you. Standing with perfect posture makes you appear slimmer, taller and younger, as well as oozing with confidence. By regularly performing the toning exercises within this book you will help realign the body, developing natural, perfect body alignment. Nowadays our posture tends to suffer as a result of too much time spent sitting at the computer or excess driving, but this way we can realign ourselves and get back to sitting and walking straight.

Question: I have never done any fitness training, and I'm now in my mid 50s. Could I still turn myself in to a fit woman?

Answer: Yes, and you will feel like a superwoman. Okay, this may sound cheesy, but it is actually a fact that many of us never realise our true abilities and how fit and strong we can be. Strength helps you take on more than just physical demands. A strong body also helps to develop a strong personality that will make you feel justified in stepping into that superwoman outfit. Plus I have a client I train who is in her late 70s and who got remarried at the age of 72 and looks incredible, so age is irrelevant.

Question: How quickly can I expect to see results?

Answer: You will see results fast. Each time you train you will notice how much stronger and fitter you are becoming. By the end of week 1 you will see the inches coming off; by the end of week 2 you can expect the total of the inches to be in double figures; and by 21 days you can easily step into a smaller sized dress. The reason being is that the strength toning workouts fire up your body's ability to burn fat, so this way not only are you sculpting your body, but you are also shifting excess body fat.

BENEFITS YOU WILL GET FROM STRENGTH TRAINING (TONING)

- ○ Strength training will keep off excess body fat.

- ○ Strength training will keep your bones strong.

- ○ Strength training will improve your posture.

- ○ Strength training will make you look and feel younger.

- ○ Strength training will increase your metabolic rate.

- ○ Strength training will help improve your balance.

- ○ Strength training will help improve your co-ordination.

- ○ Strength training will help prevent health problems.

- ○ Strength training will boost your energy levels.

- ○ Strength training will allow you to be the strongest and fittest version of you.

WHY JUST 21 DAYS

There are two reasons that 21 days work, as a timeframe. The first reason is results, and the second is habit—if you do something for 21 days, you form a habit. By doing this plan for 21 days you will see results, and this should be all you need to kick-start a healthy, fit, strong lifestyle.

Regarding the results, the great thing with fitness is that it pays you back in abundance, because every time you work out you get fitter. Each time you feel stronger, and this is such a motivational factor in living a healthy lifestyle. The more you exercise, the more energy you have, and the more energy you have, the more you want to exercise, so you can see this is a positive spiral. When you start seeing the results, including better sleep and eating well, it then simply becomes a way of life. And it is easy to see the difference.

By contrast, if we don't exercise, we have less energy, and less energy means we become even less active, and we then gain weight, leading into a downward spiral.

No matter what age, weight or fitness level, we all have the ability to begin a positive healthy spiral. And even if it is just walking for 10 minutes a day and doing a few of the exercises within my book, you will see results.

After **day 7**, you can expect to see the inches coming off, and you will notice that you have more energy.

After **day 14**, you will easily be performing more reps of each exercise, will have lost even more inches, will start seeing a difference in your body shape and will feel much fitter and more energised when you wake in the morning.

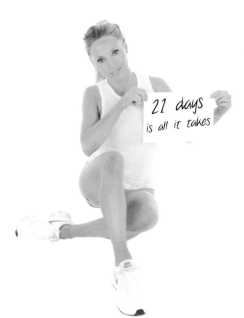

On **day 21**, you can slip into your skinny jeans or a slinky dress, as you will have lost inches all over and will be looking and feeling amazing. Even your friends and family will notice a difference.

You will be able to see the results from all the fitness training and to test and measure your success for each different section within the book. Most importantly, by day 21 you'll have formed the life-changing habit. And that's why it's 21 days!

Lucy x

2 HOW TO USE THIS BOOK

With this book I wanted to create a plan that would allow you to pick and mix the workout that you want with a clear understanding of how to put the exercise together. This would show you the progress you can make over time when mixing in different exercises, proving this book can become your permanent ongoing workout guide. With over **60** exercises provided, there is a huge abundance of mixable routines available to you so that you need never get bored.

PICK THE BODY PART YOU WANT TO TONE

Within this book are the main muscle groups of the body, particularly those areas many women want to keep toned and lifted. I have broken the body parts down into chapters covering arms, legs, abs, bust, back and butt.

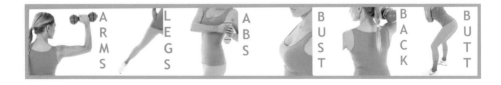

Simply select the areas that you want to tone, and choose three exercises from that specific section. I have graded each exercise, telling you how hard each move is, meaning this book suits every fitness level, from the complete beginner to the fitness enthusiast. And it will provide you with the right exercise for your current fitness level.

The grading:

✷   Suitable for beginner

✷✷   Moderate

✷✷✷   Hard

Having 10 exercises within each body part section will help stop you from getting bored, and I have carefully created the 10 moves to work that area in lots of different ranges of motion so that there is a mix of lateral movements (side to side) and twisting (rotational), as well as the most common range of motion, forwards and backwards. The benefit of having all three ranges is that this will really tighten and tone your body parts to the maximum. Many other workouts just focus on the front and back, whereas this approach will work the side and deeper muscles as well to create that beautiful, tight, sculpted, feminine body shape. And I would recommend that each couple of weeks you change routine, as this keeps the muscles guessing. You can always go back to a previous routine again, but keep mixing it up.

CREATING YOUR WORKOUT

Simply select three exercises that are suitable for your fitness level from the areas you want to tone, and then perform the recommended amount. You should aim to do this four times a week.

Also select one of the cardio workouts to do two to three times a week. These are in the cardio section, and you can choose from the:

○ 16-Minute Fat-Burning Power Walk

○ Full-Body Swimming Toning Workout

○ 15-Minute HIIT Run

○ 10 Steps to Perfect Tone Workout

CHOOSING YOUR CARDIO

The reason I have put this section in here is that I am a perfectionist, and even though many other strength training and toning books don't cover this, I wanted to include it, as I know that this will accelerate your results. It is important in fitness to always address cardio as well as toning. I have created four different easy-to-fit-in cardio workouts, and while each one is primarily aimed at weight loss and fitness, certain ones also help tone specific areas, so within each body part section I advise the best workout to go with that exercise—a bit like how a waiter would advise the best wine to complement your dinner!

EAT RIGHT

We can do all the exercise in the world, but if we are eating the wrong foods it won't work. Fitness is not just about putting on your trainers, it is also about what you eat. You need to eat yourself fit, which, trust me, can actually be delicious and tasty. If you do it right, you can still feel full and enjoy all your favourite foods, so this section of the book runs through nutrition and has some mouth-watering recipes and plenty of good nutrition tips.

MOTIVATION

This is a vital part of the book, as we must never underestimate how powerful the mind is, and we need to be able to keep positive and on track. So if you have a day where you are struggling, then quickly flip to page 172 for my prep talks and motivational triggers to help keep you on track.

HEALTH AND SAFETY

As with any exercise routine, there are always a few sensible rules we need to apply. These include:

Never exercise if you are feeling unwell.

Stop exercising if you have an injury or hurt yourself.

Always warm up properly,

and always cool down and stretch at the end of your workouts.

Always keep yourself fully hydrated.

Always perform the exercise with good form.

3 WHAT YOU NEED TO GET STARTED

YOUR KIT LIST

This section is fairly small as the great thing is that you don't need to run out and invest in lots of new fitness gear or equipment.

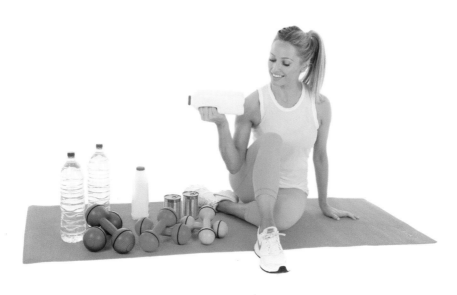

Even though this book is going to be like a multi-gym of your own, it really won't cost anything. Within the exercises we use our own body weight. For a few of the exercises I do recommend small weights, but you can use household items that will work just as well. As this book is not about bodybuilding, we do not need heavy weights. The following are the weights I suggest:

Smaller weights
1 kg or, as an equivalent, a tin of soup

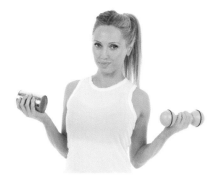

Medium weights
2 kg or plastic bottle of milk, 1 litre

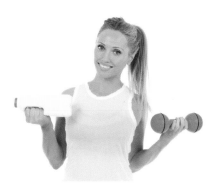

Heavier weights
3 kg or plastic water bottles, 2 litres

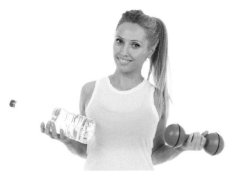

A mat is a good idea to use on the floor exercises, but alternatively you could compromise by using a thick towel.

As for your training kit, it is always a sensible idea to have a good pair of well-fitted trainers and a good sports bra. As for the rest of your kit, again you don't need to go out on a shopping spree, as leggings, tracksuit bottoms and a t-shirt are fine. However, it may be that you want to treat yourself to some funky, bright fitness gear, as this is actually a great motivator. As you can see from all my pictures in this book, I have a vast array of bright fitness clothing, because I do believe it really helps having nice clothes to work out in. But then that could be your incentive to go out and treat yourself in 21 days' time, as you will be going down a dress size or two.

21-DAY PROMISE

If you do the exercises within this book, follow the recommended cardio workout and eat well, then my promise to you is you will see amazing results. But what is more important is that you now have to promise yourself that for the next 21 days you are going to stick to the plan and have that be a genuine commitment.

So why not write out '21-day promise' on a sticky note and stick it on the fridge? Also put one into your phone or anywhere else you might look, as a constant reminder.

ORGANISATION

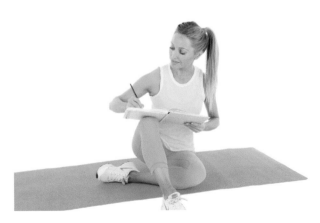

There is a great expression that is so true, which is 'fail to plan, plan to fail'. Because failing is not an option for us, we are going to be super organised and plan ahead.

Each week work out your exercises and write them down, and book in the times you are scheduled to do your workout. And plan those healthy meals. Never cancel on yourself. If it is booked in the diary, you have to do it! Remember the 21-day promise.

YOUR WARM-UP AND COOL-DOWN

Before every workout it is always important to warm up and also stretch and cool down after the workout. This is for a couple of reasons:

- It helps internally warm up your muscles and joints, the benefit of this being that it helps prevent injuries, and

- it also helps your muscles become more pliable, which means you feel more mobile and are able to perform the exercises with a bigger range of movement, which is very important in order to get the best out of each exercise.

You should always spend a couple of minutes warming up, and this can be as simple as marching on the spot or walking up and down the stairs. The important thing is to make sure you feel warm before you start. My advice is to perform all the stretches that I recommend here. At the end of your workout, just march it out for a minute or so to slowly bring your heart rate back to its pre-exercise state, and then perform the stretches again. This will help prevent any injuries and will also help realign the muscles after training.

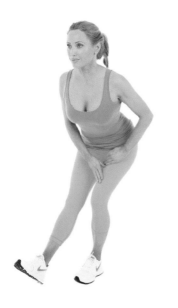

Hamstring Stretch

Standing straight, bend one leg and extend the other out straight, with heel on the floor and toes pointing up. Place both hands on the bent leg and stick your bottom out to feel the stretch along the back of the straight leg. Hold for 20 seconds on each leg.

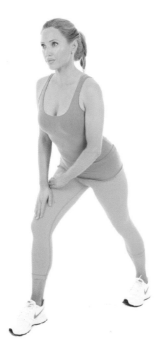

Calf Stretch

Step back with one leg, keeping the back heel down and both feet pointing forward. Rest your hands on the bent leg. Hold for 10 seconds on each leg.

Thigh Stretch

Stand with good posture. Bend one leg behind you and gently hold the foot of the bent leg, keeping the thigh close to the supporting leg. Push your hips forward to feel the stretch in the front of your thigh. Keep the supporting knee slightly bent. Hold for 10 seconds on each leg.

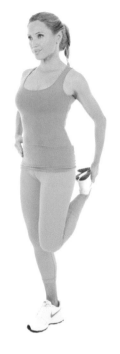

Chest Stretch

Stand with good posture. Put your arms behind you and clasp your hands, lifting your shoulders up and back to feel the stretch in the chest. Hold for 10 seconds.

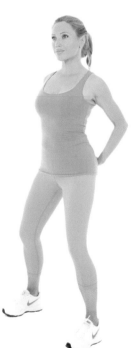

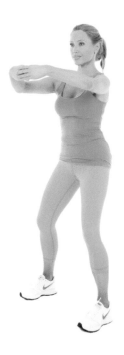

Back Stretch

Stand with good posture, keeping the knees soft and the tummy pulled in. Put your arms in front of you, clasp your hands and imagine you are hugging a big beach ball. Feel the stretch in your back. Hold for 10 seconds.

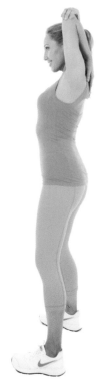

Triceps Stretch

Stand with a strong, firm, straight back, with knees slightly bent and tummy pulled in. Lift one arm up and bend it behind your head, aiming to get your hand between your shoulder blades. Put the opposite arm on the elbow of the bent arm. Hold for 10 seconds.

Part 2

4 ABS

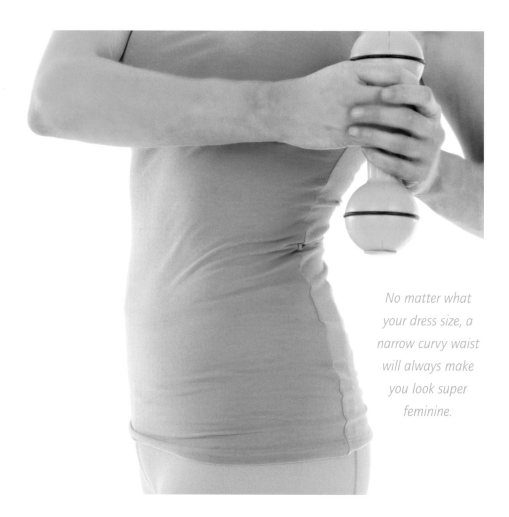

No matter what your dress size, a narrow curvy waist will always make you look super feminine.

Having a flat belly is pretty much the thing at the top of most women's wish list! Especially come holiday season when you bare your midriff by the pool, and it can be the difference between hiding your tummy under a one piece or feeling proud and wearing a bikini.

But the abdominals are more complex than just having what is often referred to as a desired six-pack. Even though our body shapes and where we store fat is different, this is one area where most people find it's the hardest to shift fat, and it can also be the first place fat heads. And in this context we often hear the expression ‚middle-age spread', which is largely due to the process I have mentioned before in which the muscles in our body begin slowing down and become less metabolically active, but remember the good news is we can reverse this by doing exercise, as this immediately makes them fire up again. So this can help melt away that excess fat around the middle, such as the dreaded muffin top or love handles that protrude over your waistband.

As we age it is very important to aim to keep our waist measurement within a healthy range, as carrying too much weight around our abdominals can have an effect on our health. This fat on the tummy is referred to as visceral fat, which is located between internal organs and the torso, as opposed to fat such as that on the butt, known as subcutaneous fat, which is found underneath the skin. Abdominal fat (visceral fat) can be strongly associated with type 2 diabetes. So even more than the way you look in a bikini, this should be a good incentive to aim to keep your waist measurement within a healthy range. Your health can be at risk if this exceeds 31.5 inches and at an even higher risk if over 34.5 inches.

But if you measure yours now and find it is beyond that range, do not panic, as this book is going to help you easily get it back within a healthy range. You'll be able to watch those inches come down in the next 21 days.

4

Please note that if you do need to lose excess tummy fat it is important that you not only do the cardio workout I recommend, but also eat well, as bad fat will head straight to those abs!

The abdominals are made up of three main muscle groups. The deepest abdominal muscle is known as the *transversus abdominis*, and this is like a corset that wraps horizontally around your torso. This muscle helps with posture and balance, looks after your back, and helps shape your waist. Then sitting on top of this are what are known as your *internal* and *external obliques*. These are what create a lovely, narrow, curvy waist, and these muscles help you rotate and twist from side to side. The outermost muscle is the *rectus abdominis*, which runs vertically down the front of your torso and allows you to bend forwards and backwards. This one is often referred to as a six-pack, but it is actually just one long muscle with a tiny central separation which then enables the muscles to separate in pregnancy, allowing the baby to grow.

This is why it is especially important for women who have children to understand the muscles and work all three, not just the top one, as we need to strengthen and tone your deep muscles so that the top muscles can lie flat.

But the secret to a flat tummy (which we can all have) is strength toning, cardio, and eating the right food.

THE BENEFITS OF TONING THIS AREA

- You will notice that your waistband starts to feel looser.

- You will have a stronger back.

- You will find you stand with better posture.

- You will find that muffin tops and love handles disappear.

- You will improve your health and fitness.

- You will pack a bikini for your summer holidays.

For the cardio section I recommend a couple workouts here. You could either do the 16-Minute Fat-Burning Powerwalk (page 149) or the 15-Minute HIIT Run (page 151). Both these workouts will help to strip off excess belly fat, melting away that spare tyre.

10 ABDOMINAL-TONING MOVES

Each exercise has a suggested number of repetitions (e.g., the amount of times you perform the exercise) along with how many sets you do. As you become fitter each week, you can adapt the workout. For example, for the first week do the recommended amounts for a beginner, then progress to intermediate the next week, and then advanced the final week.

Additionally, next to the name of each exercise is a star, and this provides you with a grade as to how hard the exercise is:

✳   Light

✳✳   Moderate

✳✳✳   Hard

Half Star ★★

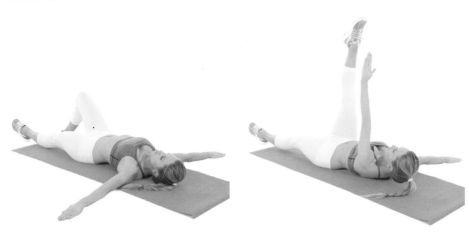

Step 1: Lie face up on your mat with both your arms out to your sides and in line with your shoulders. Extend one leg out straight and bend the other leg, placing the foot flat on the floor.

Step 2: Move the bent leg to a straight upwards position, extending it fully. Now bring the opposite hand up towards the foot. Hold for a second, and then, keeping the leg in the same position, lower just your hand back down to the starting position. It is important that throughout this exercise you keep your tummy muscles pulled in, and aim to keep the extended leg as still as possible.

Beginner:	10-12 reps, 2 sets
Intermediate:	18-20 reps, 3 sets
Advanced:	20-24 reps, 4 sets

Killer Curves ★★★

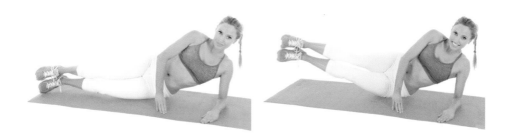

Step 1: Lie on your side, leaning on that side's forearm, with your top arm in front and your fingers just gently touching the floor. (Don't put too much pressure on them, because then the arms do the work instead of the abs, so keep the pressure off.) Your legs should be stacked, with knees slightly bent.

Step 2: Now fully engage your abdominal muscles and aim to lift your legs off the floor, focusing so that the lift comes from your waist. Hold and then slowly lower to your starting position. Repeat one set on one side and then change to do the other side.

Beginner: 6-8 reps, 2 sets
Intermediate: 12-14 reps, 3 sets
Advanced: 16-20 reps, 4 sets

Wonder Waist ★★

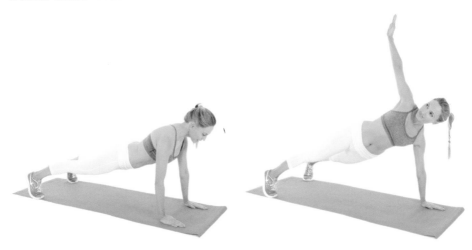

Step 1: Start with your hands and feet on your mat in a fully extended plank position, with your tummy muscles pulled in.

Step 2: Now gently extend one arm up and out to the side, aiming to point your fingers directly up towards the ceiling. Hold for a second, and then return to your starting position. Then work on the opposite side.

Beginner: 10-12 reps, 2 sets
Intermediate: 16-18 reps, 3 sets
Advanced: 20-26 reps, 4 sets

Kneeling Ab Toner ★★

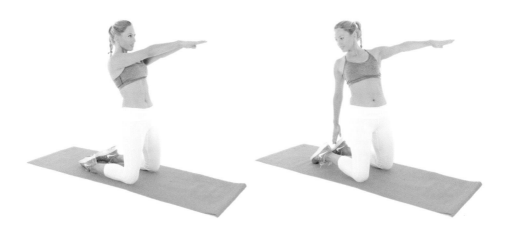

Step 1: Kneeling on your mat, fully engage your tummy muscles and lean back slightly. Extend both arms directly out in front of you.

Step 2: Keeping your tummy muscles pulled in, aim to reach one hand around to touch the heel of your foot. Hold for a second, and then slowly come back to the starting position. Then repeat on the opposite side.

Beginner:	8-10 reps, 2 sets
Intermediate:	16-18 reps, 3 sets
Advanced:	20-24 reps, 4 sets

Facedown Ab Crunch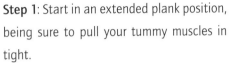

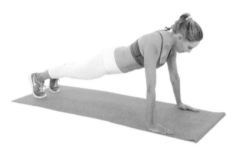

Step 1: Start in an extended plank position, being sure to pull your tummy muscles in tight.

Step 2: In a slow, controlled move, bring your knee over towards the opposite hip, keeping the shoulders in line with your wrists. Hold and then bring the leg back to your starting position. Repeat using the opposite leg.

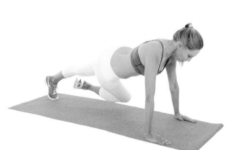

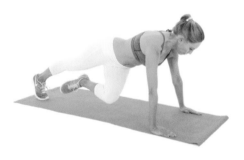

Beginner:	14-18 reps, 2 sets
Intermediate:	18-20 reps, 3 sets
Advanced:	30 reps, 4 sets

Ab Makeover ✿✿

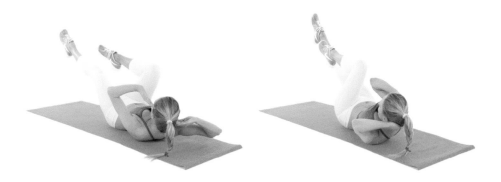

Step 1: Lie face up on your mat, with your fingertips touching the side of your head and one leg bent and the other extended. Raise both legs off the floor, making sure you keep you tummy muscles fully engaged.

Step 2: Now take your elbow over towards your opposite knee. Hold, and then change to the other side by bringing the other leg into a bent position and extending the other. Aim to get the opposite elbow over towards the bent knee. Keep rotating from side to side.

Beginner: 12-14 reps, 2 sets
Intermediate: 18-20 reps, 3 sets
Advanced: 30 reps, 4 sets

Basic Flat Tummy Lift ⭐

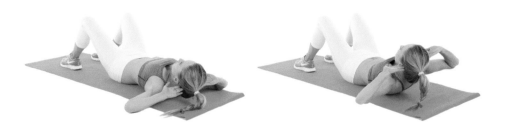

Step 1: Lie face up on your mat with your knees bent and tummy pulled in. Bend your arms, touching your fingertips to your ears.

Step 2: Now pull in your tummy muscles and aim to lift your head and shoulders off the floor by several inches. Hold, and then slowly lower back down. Keep repeating.

Beginner: 10-12 reps, 2 sets
Intermediate: 18-22 reps, 3 sets
Advanced: 30 reps, 4 sets

Bikini Lift ✿✿✿

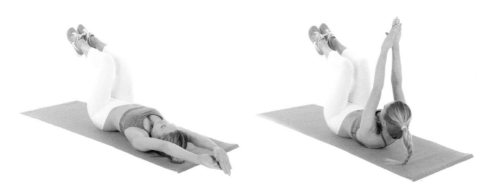

Step 1: Lie face up, with your knees bent and feet off the floor. Aim to get your feet in line with your knees and your knees over the line of your hips at a 90-degree angle. Extend both arms directly overhead on the floor, with your palms facing up.

Step 2: Now slowly lift your head and shoulders off the floor, keeping your arms straight, trying to get them in line with your shoulders (constantly keeping your tummy pulled in). Hold, and then slowly lower back down to your starting position.

Beginner:	6-8 reps, 2 sets
Intermediate:	12-14 reps, 3 sets
Advanced:	25 reps, 4 sets

Ab Climb ★★

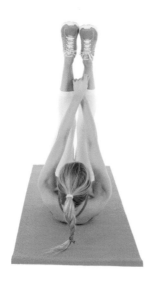

Step 1: Lie face up with your legs fully extended, trying to get your feet in line with your hips.

Step 2: Imagine you have a piece of rope wrapped around your feet, and the rope is hanging directly down. Now lift your head and shoulders off the floor, extending your arms up, and imagine you are holding on to the rope. Now imagine your hands are climbing up the rope, and try to get as close as possible to your feet, keeping your head and shoulders off the floor.

Beginner:	20 reps, 2 sets
Intermediate:	30 reps, 3 sets
Advanced:	40 reps, 4 sets

Waist Inch Loss Twist ✦✦

Step 1: Lie face up with both legs extended straight up, feet in line with your hips, your arms extended out to your sides and in line with your shoulders, and your palms facing up. If you have a sensitive back, you can also place your hands under your bottom

Step 2: Pull in your tummy muscles tight and slowly lower your legs several inches to one side, still keeping your feet over the line of your hips. Hold, and then slowly bring the legs back to the centre before lowering them several inches to the other side. All the time it is important to keep your abdominals pulled in.

For an easier variation, you can also keep your legs bent.

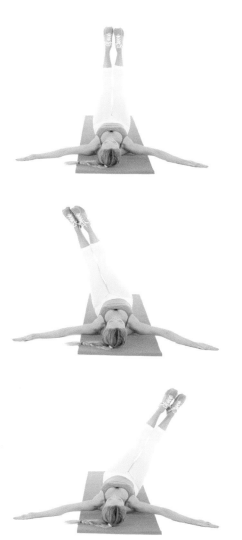

4

Beginner:	6-8 reps, 2 sets
Intermediate:	12-14 reps, 3 sets
Advanced:	16-20 reps, 4 sets

FREQUENTLY ASKED QUESTIONS: ABDOMINALS

Question: I often get a sore neck when I am doing sit-ups; is there an alternative?

Answer: Absolutely. You can tone abdominal muscles without doing sit-ups. Try pulling in your tummy muscles and holding for 10 seconds; do this several times a day. Plus the exercises within this section that will help build up your abdominal strength are:

- Killer Curves,
- Wonder Waist,
- Kneeling Ab Toner,
- Facedown Ab Crunch and
- Waist Inch Loss Twist.

You will find that by doing these exercises you will tone and build up endurance and strength in your tummy muscles, and this means you should soon be able to do any abdominal exercise without getting a sore neck.

You should also always avoid pulling on your head when you are doing abdominal exercises so you don't strain your neck.

Question: Will doing abdominal exercise help to strengthen my back?

Answer: Yes, and this is one of the main reasons we should all be doing them, not just to have those fab abs in a bikini. Having strong tummy muscles helps to protect your back and also promotes good posture, so the stronger your abs are, the better back health you will have.

Question: I am a typical apple shape, and my waist is not very defined. Is there any specific exercise I can do to help get a curvier waist?

Answer: The way you can help to draw in your waist is to focus on exercises that have a slight rotation in the move, as this will engage your oblique muscles which crisscross around your waist, and the more toned these are, the narrower your waist will become. In this section the exercises that will really help in that are the Waist Toner, the Ab Makeover and the Waist Inch Loss Twist.

MEASURE YOUR PROGRESS

Abdominal fitness

Each week you will find that as the abdominals become stronger, you are able to perform more repetitions of each move. Measure your starting abdominal fitness by doing the Basic Flat Tummy Lift and seeing how many you can do in 30 seconds with good form. Make a note of this, and then redo the measurement every two weeks.

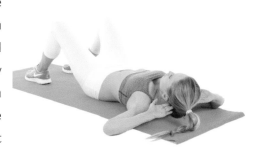

Abdominal measurements

This is an area where you will notice some dramatic results, especially if you are focusing on eating a healthy diet and doing some cardio workouts. Using a tape measure, measure at the narrowest part of your waist. Avoid pulling in your tummy muscles, just let them be relaxed. Make a note of your measurement. Measure your waist every two weeks.

ABDOMINAL BEAUTY TIP

The abs can be one area where stretch marks appear, so this DIY skin smoothing treatment is to help reduce the appearance of them.

Ingredients:

1 tablespoon ground coffee
1 teaspoon honey
1 tablespoon vitamin E oil
Mix together into a paste, and apply to your tummy, gently rubbing it in. Then wrap some cling film around your waist, and leave it on for 15-20 minutes. Then rinse off thoroughly.

4

5 BOTTOM

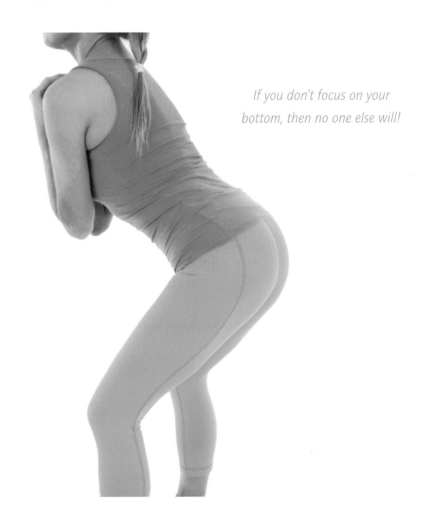

If you don't focus on your bottom, then no one else will!

So whether you call it your butt, derrière, bottom, or glutes, this is one muscle group that pays dividends when it's super toned. These are some of the biggest muscles in your body, which means if you keep this area toned, your body burns more calories.

A sculpted butt gives you a great curvy silhouette, and toning this section of muscles in the gluteus is easy when you know just how to lift, sculpt and shape.

The bottom has three main muscles that help to shape it, and many workouts just focus on working the one muscle called the *gluteus maximus*, which is the biggest, but the other two, known as the *gluteus minimus* and *gluteus medius*, need to be trained also. So you must target this area from three angles, and this can take your butt from a flat peach to a perfect, rounded peach.

In this day and age this is one muscle in the body that we do tend to spend a lot of time just sitting on rather than exercising, either due to having extra workloads in the office seated at a desk, sitting in the car stuck in traffic, or simply being planted on the sofa. All the more reason to decide to stop having a 'chair bottom', and change it to a 'perfect bottom'.

We naturally engage the main muscle in the butt, the gluteus maximus, by doing simple moves like walking, going up and down the stairs, or coming from a seated position to a standing position. But very rarely do we do all that we need in our daily activities, and that includes side moves and rotations from the hip.

The exercises within this section will combat this, and there's a great cardio workout that I would recommend to complement toning your butt: the 10 Steps to Perfect Tone Workout. You can see the full workout on page 153.

5

THE BENEFITS OF TONING THIS AREA

- You will notice that your bottom becomes more pert.

- You will notice you have better posture, as a stronger bottom helps spinal alignment.

- You will increase the amount of calories your body burns on an hourly rate.

- You will feel super sexy in your skinny jeans.

- You will reduce the appearance of cellulite.

- You will notice that your bottom feels firmer.

10 BOTTOM-TONING MOVES

Each exercise has a suggested number of repetitions (e.g., the amount of times you perform the exercise) as well as the number of sets you do. As you become fitter each week, you can adapt the workout. For example for the first week do the recommended amounts for a beginner, then progress to intermediate the next week, and then to advanced the final week.

Additionally, there is a star by the name of each exercise, and this provides you with a grade as to how hard the exercise is:

⭐   Light

⭐⭐   Moderate

⭐⭐⭐   Hard

Perfect Peach ✻

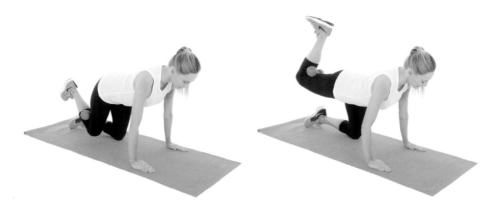

Step 1: Taking either a hand weight or a bottle of water, get down on your mat on all fours. Place the object in the fold of your knee, and lift the lower leg slightly to secure a firm grip.

Step 2: With your tummy muscles fully engaged and belly button tight to your spine, lift the leg with the weight up to hip height. Be sure to squeeze tight into the bottom. Hold for a second, and then slowly lower to your starting position. Complete full reps on one side before switching legs.

Beginner: 12-14 reps, 2 sets
Intermediate: 20-24 reps, 3 sets
Advanced: 30 reps, 4 sets

Straight-Leg Butt Lift ✳

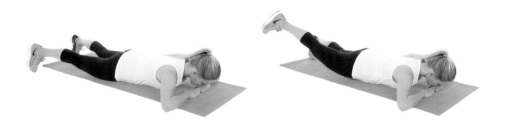

Step 1: Lie facedown on your mat, with your arms bent in front. Keep one leg straight so that your heel is in line with your hip, and take the other leg out to the side to a 45-degree angle.

Step 2: Just working the leg that's out to the side, firstly pull in your abdominals and then lift your leg off the floor and hold. Slowly lower to the starting position. Complete full reps on one leg and then switch legs.

Beginner: 15 reps, 2 sets
Intermediate: 20 reps, 3 sets
Advanced: 30 reps, 4 sets

5

Designer Derrière ✿✿

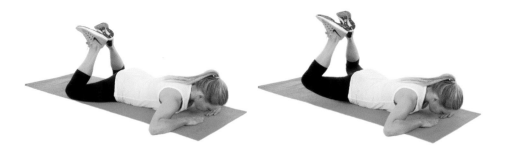

Step 1: Lie facedown on your mat, with your arms bent and hands firmly on the ground. Keep looking facedown. Bend your knees and bring your heels together, keeping toes and knees turned out. Your feet should be flexed so that your toes are pointing forwards.

Step 2: Pull in your abdominals and squeeze tight into your bottom, lifting both your thighs off the ground. Hold for a second, and then slowly lower back to your starting position.

Beginner: 10-12 reps, 2 sets
Intermediate: 18-20 reps, 3 sets
Advanced: 20-24 reps, 4 sets

Skinny Jeans Squeeze ✿✿

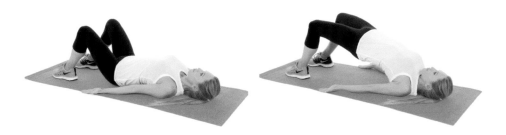

Step 1: Lie face up on your mat, with your knees bent and arms out to your side, palms facing up.

Step 2: Now push your hips up as high as you can by squeezing tight into your bottom. Try to avoid pushing through your hands (this is why I recommend palms up) so that all the work will be coming from the bottom. Hold, and then slowly lower back down to your starting position.

Beginner:	12-16 reps, 2 sets
Intermediate:	20-24 reps, 3 sets
Advanced:	26-30 reps, 4 sets

5

Lying Butt Sculptor ★★

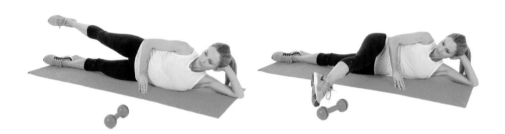

Step 1: Lie on your side with a weight or bottle of water placed out in front of you about 10 inches away from your hip. Position the floor-side arm so that it is bent and supporting your head. Bend your top arm and rest the hand gently in front for support.

Step 2: Lift your top leg slightly, pull your tummy muscles in tight. Now very slowly bring your foot over to the weight. Hold, and then slowly return back to the starting position. Complete all reps on one leg and then switch legs.

Beginner: 12-14 reps, 2 sets
Intermediate: 18-20 reps, 3 sets
Advanced: 26-30 reps, 4 sets

Squat ★★

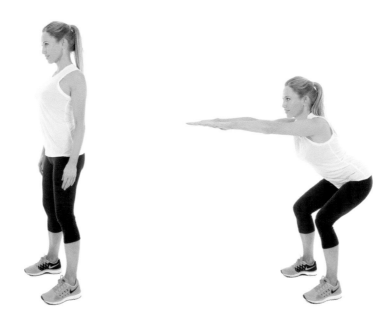

Step 1: Start with your feet hip-width distance apart, standing with good posture.

Step 2: Now slowly bend through your knees, sticking your bottom back as far as you can as if you were sitting into a chair. Simultaneously bring your arms straight out in front to shoulder height. Do not let your knees come over the line of your toes. Then slowly push back up to your starting position.

5

Beginner:	12-14 reps, 2 sets
Intermediate:	20-26 reps, 3 sets
Advanced:	30 reps, 4 sets

Brazilian Butt Squat Drop ✿✿✿

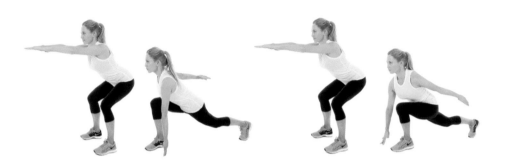

Step 1: Start in a deep squat position, with your bottom sticking out and arms extended in front. Now step one leg behind. At the same time, move the arm on the same side as the back leg down, touching the fingertips to the ground. Hold.

Step 2: Now push straight back up to your deep squat starting position. Then step the other leg back and touch the other hand to the ground. Then come back to your starting position. Keep alternating the leg you step back for the required reps.

Beginner:	6-8 reps, 2 sets
Intermediate:	10-12 reps, 3 sets
Advanced:	16-20 reps, 4 sets

Firm Butt Drop ✿✿✿

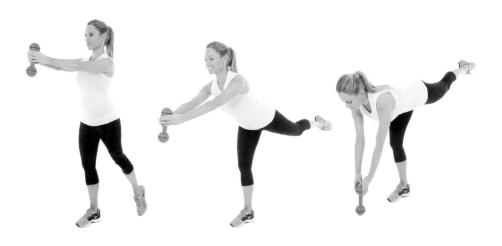

Step 1: Stand in a split stance, with one foot behind the other and your arms directly in front of you, holding on to a weight or a water bottle.

Step 2: Pulling in your tummy muscles tight to your spine, lift your leg up behind you, and slowly take the weight down towards the ground. Hold for a second, and then ease back up to the fully extended starting position.

Beginner: 6-8 reps, 2 sets
Intermediate: 10-12 reps, 3 sets
Advanced: 16 reps, 4 sets

5

Ballerina's Butt ★★

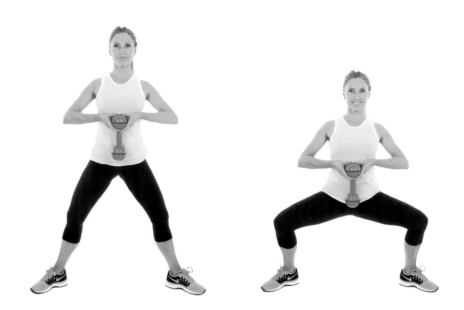

Step 1: Stand with your feet wide apart and your toes turned out to a 45-degree angle. Your upper body should be perfectly straight, holding on to your hand weight or water bottle, with your elbows bent out to your side, and the weight directly in the middle of your body.

Step 2: Bend your knees out to the side, aiming to get your hips in line with your knees. Do not let the knees go over the line of your toes. Hold, and then slowly push back up. Be sure to keep your upper body perfectly straight as your perform this move.

Beginner: 12-14 reps, 2 sets
Intermediate: 16-20 reps, 3 sets
Advanced: 30 reps, 4 sets

Curtsey ✿✿

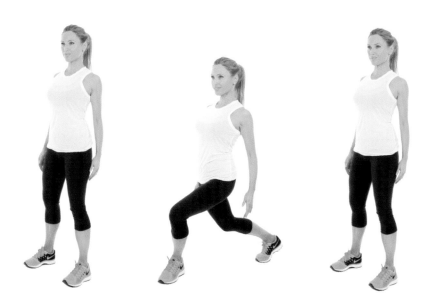

Step 1: Stand with good posture and your feet shoulder-width distance apart, with shoulders pulled back and tummy muscles pulled in.

Step 2: Now step one leg back and behind the line of the front foot, as if you are curtseying. Still keeping the upper body straight, bend low, making sure the front knee does not go over the line of the toes. Hold, and then push back up to your starting position. Then curtsey back on the other leg, alternating for the required reps.

Beginner: 8-10 reps, 2 sets
Intermediate: 16-18 reps, 3 sets
Advanced: 30 reps, 4 sets

FREQUENTLY ASKED QUESTIONS: BOTTOM

Question: Is it possible to lift and improve the shape of your bottom?

Answer: Yes, by targeting the three muscles we can lift and tone the butt, and in this book we cover all three muscles so that you can get that perfect rounded butt.

Question: I work really long hours and am sitting at a desk sometimes for eight hours a day, and I have really noticed that my bottom has become bigger; what can I do about this?

Answer: The Office Backside is a real problem for two reasons: 1) when we sit down for long periods of time our body starts to reduce the amount of calories we burn, so if we are seated at a desk for long periods our metabolism begins to slow down. So a quick tip to address this is to make sure you get up from your desk every 20 minutes, even if it just to get a glass of water. This will help to keep your body burning calories at a higher rate; and 2) being sedentary can reduce our energy levels, meaning we are less likely to exercise. So make it a rule that in your lunch hour you always head out of the office for a quick powerwalk, as this will fire up your glutes and give them a quick workout.

MEASURE YOUR PROGRESS

Bottom fitness

It's good to measure and see how much you have improved your muscular strength and endurance in your bottom with time.

I recommend that you perform a squat as shown here and see how many seconds you can hold it for whilst still maintaining good form. It is very important that you do not let the line of the knees come over the line of your toes, so focus on keeping the bottom sticking out.

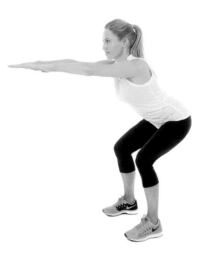

Only do this test once you are fully warmed up. Because this is tough, have a stopwatch on hand and make a note of how many seconds you were able to hold it for. And then redo this test every couple of weeks.

Bottom measurements

Wrap a tape measure around the widest part of your bottom, or alternatively you can measure it in line with your pubic bone, but however you do it, be sure to always measure at the exact same point every couple of weeks.

The other great way to measure your success is simply to step into your tightest skinny jeans. Noticing they have a smoother fit should put a smile on your face.

BOTTOM BEAUTY TIP

Polish your posterior weekly with this DIY scrub of mine.

Ingredients:
1 tablespoon olive oil
1 teaspoon Demerara sugar

Simply mix together to form a paste, and then apply to your glutes and massage in well. Then shower off, and always apply a good moisturiser.

6   LEGS

Have a good legs day,
every day.

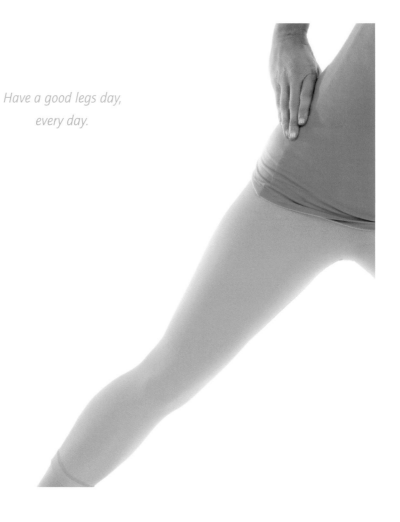

Having the perfect pins gives you the freedom to wear anything, from shorts to your skinny jeans, and even to slip into a little black dress that will showcase your legs.

Your legs are already far from lazy, as you use them from the minute you jump out of bed, rushing to catch the bus for your commute, walking around the shops or running up and down the stairs. So we do engage these muscles naturally within our daily activities, but—and there is always a but—the movement we mainly do is a forwards motion. This helps to engage the muscles that are located down the front and back of the leg—quadriceps, front thigh, and hamstring, back of the thighs—YET the side muscles in the legs which help tighten, shape and give you those gorgeous sexy pins are often neglected. These muscles are known as the *adductors* (inner thighs) and *abductors* (outer thighs).

This is why, when it comes to doing strength toning exercises, it is important to do a mixture of movements that not only work your legs through a forwards and backwards motion, but also through a sideways motion, as this will nip and tone your inner and outer thighs. So come the warm weather you will have the confidence to have a high hemline on your skirt.

The legs can be an area that cellulite (sometimes referred to as cottage cheese thighs or orange peel because of its dimple effect) can sneak onto, but with healthy eating and a mix of cardio and toning, you can help to reduce the effects of cellulite. So don't worry if you can relate to this, as with these workouts it will be time to wave goodbye to dimply thighs.

6

THE BENEFITS OF TONING THIS AREA

○ You will help reduce cellulite.

○ You will lose inches on your thighs.

○ Your legs will look super toned.

○ You will want to be wearing a skirt.

○ You will have perfect pins.

○ You will have better flexibility.

For cardio exercise I recommend the 16-Minute Fat-Burning Powerwalk, as this will also strengthen, tone and sculpt through your thighs, butt and lower legs muscles. See page 149 for the workout.

10 LEG-TONING MOVES

Each exercise has a suggested number of repetitions (e.g., the amount of times you perform the exercise) as well as how many sets you do. As you become fitter each week, you can adapt the workout. For example, for the first week do the recommended amounts for a beginner, then progress to intermediate the next week, and then to advanced the final week.

Additionally, the stars next to each exercise allow you to grade how hard the exercise is:

★   Light

★★   Moderate

★★★ Hard

Kick It to Tone It ✭

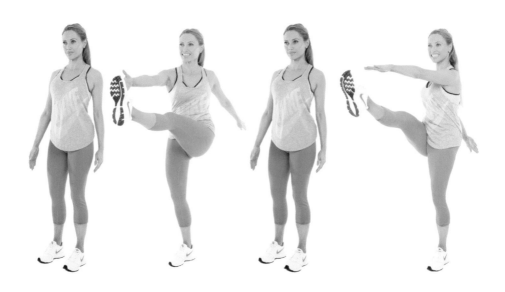

Step 1: Stand with your feet hip-width distance apart and your arms relaxed down by your sides. Keep your tummy muscles pulled in.

Step 2: Kick one leg straight out in front. Extend your opposite arm and try to touch your extended foot. Then return to your starting position. Now work the opposite arm and leg. At all times be sure to keep your back straight and your abdominals pulled in tight.

Beginner: 12-16 reps, 2 sets
Intermediate: 20-24 reps, 3 sets
Advanced: 40 reps, 4 sets

Love Your Legs Lunge ★★

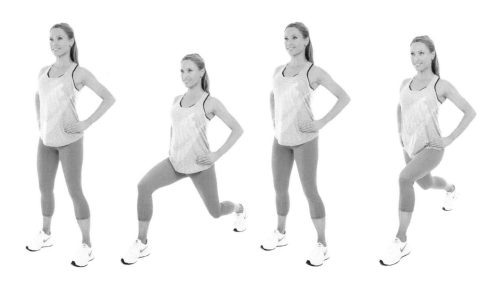

Step 1: Stand in a stance that is slightly wider than shoulder-width distance apart and place your hands on your hips, with your shoulders pulled back and chest lifted.

Step 2: Now step forward into a lunge position. Do not let the front knee come over the line of your toes, and keep the knee of your back leg pointing down towards the ground, with your upper body straight. Hold, and then push back to your starting position. Alternate from leg to leg for the required reps.

Beginner: 10-12 reps, 2 sets
Intermediate: 14-18 reps, 3 sets
Advanced: 30 reps, 4 sets

Perfect Pin Lunge ⭐⭐

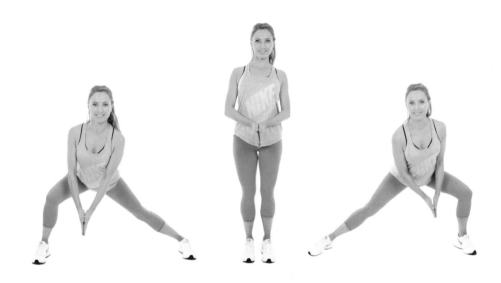

Step 1: Start with one leg extended straight out to the side and the other leg bent. Press your palms together, with fingers pointing down, keeping tummy pulled in.

Step 2: Now push off from your bent leg, coming up to a standing position with the palms still pressed together. Then lunge straight out to the opposite side. Keep alternating from side to side for the required reps.

Beginner: 12-14 reps, 2 sets
Intermediate: 20-24 reps, 3 sets
Advanced: 30 reps, 4 sets

I Love Shoes Lift   ⭐

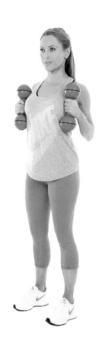 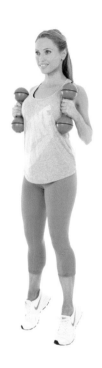

Step 1: Stand with your feet hip-width distance apart. Hold on to your weights, with your arms bent and the weights tucked in by your sides and tummy pulled in.

Step 2: Keeping the body straight, slowly lift both your heels off the floor until you are balancing on your toes. Be sure to pull in your tummy muscles at the same time, as this will help with balance and stability. Hold, and then slowly lower the heels back down to the ground.

6

Beginner: 14-18 reps, 2 sets
Intermediate: 20-24 reps, 3 sets
Advanced: 30 reps, 4 sets

Inner Thigh Ultimate Toner ★

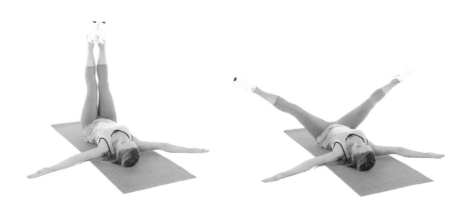

Step 1: Lie face up on your mat, with your arms out to your sides and in line with your shoulders. Extend your legs straight up, directly over the line of your hips.

Step 2: Now in a slow and controlled manner take your legs out to either side. Hold at the farthest range of motion they will reach, and then slowly draw back up to the starting position.

Beginner:	16-20 reps, 2 sets
Intermediate:	30 reps, 3 sets
Advanced:	40 reps, 4 sets

Catwalk Pins ★★

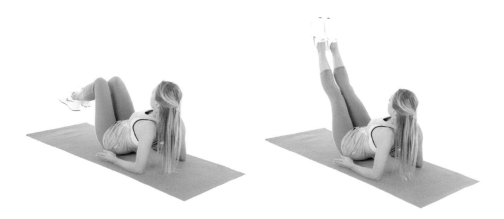

Step 1: Come to a sitting position on your mat. Rest back on your forearms, with your hands pointing forwards, knees bent and feet lifted off the floor and tummy pulled in.

Step 2: Keeping the tummy muscles pulled in, straighten your legs, hold and then bend back to the starting position.

Beginner: 12-14 reps, 2 sets
Intermediate: 20-22 reps, 3 sets
Advanced: 30 reps, 4 sets

Two-Step Lean Legs Lift ✹✹✹

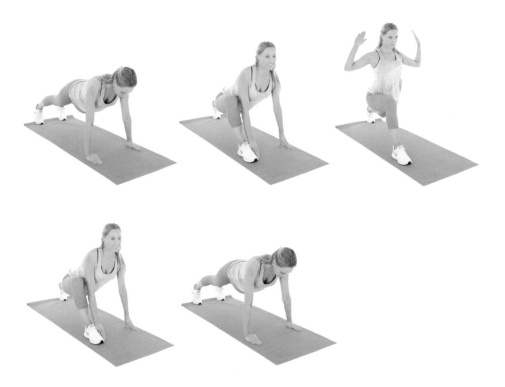

Step 1: Start in a fully extended plank position, with your tummy pulled in.

Step 2: Now step one foot towards your hand. Hold, and then come up so that your upper body is straight, with both your arms bent and extended out to your sides. Hold, and then bring your hands back down to the ground. Then step the foot back. Alternate legs for the required reps.

Beginner: 4 reps, 2 sets
Intermediate: 8 reps, 3 sets
Advanced: 12 reps, 4 sets

Rainbow Inner and Outer Thigh Lift ✿✿

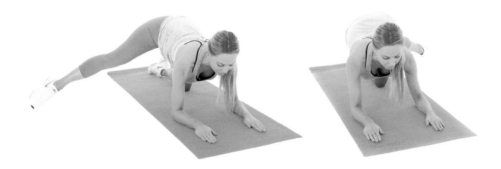

Step 1: Kneel on your mat, with forearms on the floor, palms facing down and fingers pointing forwards. Extend one leg out to your side.

Step 2: Fully engage your tummy muscles and raise your extended leg off the floor. Lift your leg behind you, up and over, as if you are drawing a rainbow. Try to touch your foot down on the other side. Hold, and then bring the leg back to your starting position. Complete all reps on one leg before switching to the other leg.

Beginner: 8-10 reps, 2 sets
Intermediate: 14-16 reps, 3 sets
Advanced: 20 reps, 4 sets

6

Thigh Shaper ★

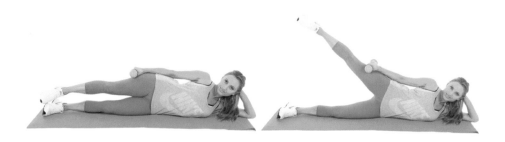

Step 1: Lie on your side. Rest a weight on the top leg. Your body should be in a straight line, with your bottom arm bent and head resting on your hand.

Step 2: Now slowly lift your top leg, still keeping the weight pressed to the leg. Hold at the highest point. Make sure that you don't turn the leg out from the hip. Your toes should stay pointing forwards. Hold, and then slowly lower to your starting position.

Beginner: 14-16 reps, 2 sets
Intermediate: 18-20 reps, 3 sets
Advanced: 30 reps, 4 sets

Thigh Inch Loss Lift ★★★

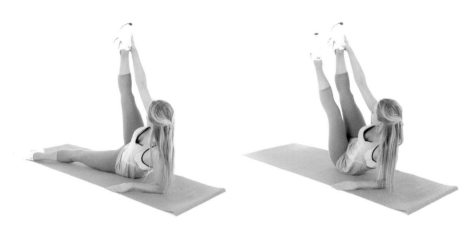

Step 1: Get down on your mat with one leg on the floor and your upper body propped up on your forearm. Extend the other leg directly up and hold on to your foot using the same-side arm.

Step 2: Using your inner thigh, lift the lower leg from the floor. Try to bring it up to your extended leg. Hold, and then slowly lower all the way back down. Complete all reps on one leg, and then change position to work the opposite leg for the required reps.

Beginner:	6-8 reps, 2 sets
Intermediate:	10-12 reps, 3 sets
Advanced:	18-20 reps, 4 sets

6

FREQUENTLY ASKED QUESTIONS: LEGS

Question: I have quite bad cellulite on my legs; is there anything I can do about this?

Answer: Cellulite is an accumulation of toxins and fatty deposits that get trapped in the cells beneath the skin; this is why we can have cellulite not just on our legs but also on other areas such as arms and the tummy. We can very easily reduce cellulite. The most effective and easiest ways are drinking more water to help flush away toxins; eating fresh, clean and healthy foods; and most importantly doing a mix of cardio workouts and strength training exercises. The cellulite will soon start to disappear.

Question: What is the best way to get thinner thighs?

Answer: This comes down to toning the inside and outside of your thighs. You will find plenty of exercises to choose from in this section, and powerwalking (plus a healthy diet) is a great way to tone and sculpt your legs. With every stride you take, you engage your thigh muscles and also help lift the butt, so this way you can easily get those thinner thighs. Exercises I recommend to work deep into those inner thigh muscles are the Thigh Inch Loss Lift and the Inner Thigh Ultimate Toner.

MEASURE YOUR PROGRESS

Leg fitness

Each week you will find that as the legs become stronger, you are able to perform more repetitions of each move. Measure your starting leg fitness by doing the Basic Lunge and seeing how many you can do before your legs start to feel challenged. Make a note of this number and then redo the measurement every two weeks.

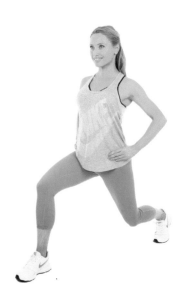

Thigh measurements

The legs will tone up fast when doing these workouts, and you will notice some exciting results, especially if you are focusing on eating a healthy diet and doing some cardio workouts. Find the midpoint between the lower part of the glutes and the back of the knee – the widest part of the thigh – and measure this section with a tape measure. Make a note of your measurement and then take this measurement every two weeks.

LEG BEAUTY TIP

The legs can look better instantly with a great suntan, and the best way to achieve this is with a good fake tan. So give your legs a va-va-voom treatment by applying a generous amount of self-tanning lotion. But to get the best results for this, first try this special leg body scrub of mine.

Ingredients:

1 cup brewed green tea, lukewarm

1 tablespoon sugar

2 tablespoons freshly grated ginger

Mix all these ingredients into a bowl, and then apply the mixture generously to your legs. Massage it in with an upwards circular movement. Once fully rubbed in, rinse off, and then apply your self-tanning lotion. You will wake the next day with beautiful, bronzed goddess legs.

6

7 BUST

Whatever our age,
we can still have a pert bust.

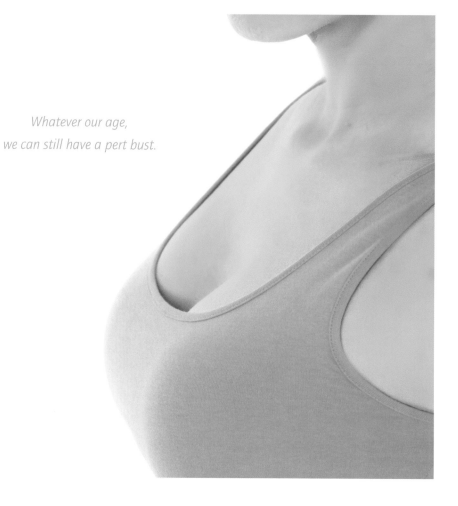

Exercise really is the fountain of youth, because if we do the right exercises, we can slow down the aging process, keep the body sculpted and keep everything firm and lifted.

The bust is one of the major areas in question, and as a female trainer, I was keen to develop a range of exercises to tackle just that. So I created a simple two-move workout as a 14-day challenge, and I put this on my YouTube channel, and within less than a year, over a quarter of a million women were taking part in the challenge. I received so many lovely comments from followers on how this had helped to lift their busts.

As always, the more we understand the body, the clearer it becomes how exercise really does work, why it is so effective and how we can naturally give you that bust lift without having to go under the knife.

So let me introduce to you *Cooper's ligaments*, which are thin collections of connective tissues that lift the bust. They are attached to your collarbone and the underlying connective tissue of the major chest muscles known as the *pectorals*. A good visualisation for this is to picture your Cooper's ligament as a bra strap. If you have a loose bra strap it will not support or lift your bust, whereas if you tighten that bra strap, it will instantly lift your bust, giving you volume and a fuller cleavage. Well, we can do this with exercise by tightening and toning your Cooper's ligament (which is what all the exercises within this section will do).

The bust is made up of two major muscles: the *pectoralis major* and *pectoralis minor*, as well as many smaller muscles. These muscles lie underneath the breast tissue and on the breastbone, and they connect to the humerus (the arm bone closest to your shoulder joint). Your chest plays a major part in helping to bring your arms across your body and your shoulders forward.

This is an area where if we don't apply regular toning exercises we start to lose definition, shape and tone, yet these exercises I have created here will turn that all around, and in less than 21 days you can expect to see your bust lift and become more pert. As with each body part, I do also recommend a good cardio exercise to combine with the toning, as this will double your results. Racket sports such as tennis or even netball are good, and the other great bust-lifting aerobic move is (you guessed it, there's a clue in the name) the breaststroke for the swimming workout.

THE BENEFITS OF TONING THIS AREA

○ You will notice that your bust becomes more pert.

○ You will notice that you have better upper-body posture.

○ Your will feel stronger through your upper body.

○ You will feel amazing when wearing low-cut tops.

○ You will notice your shoulders becoming more sculpted.

○ You will want to swap your old swimsuit for a flash new bikini.

○ You will be amazed by your progress.

So here are the 10 exercises for you to choose from to lift your bust naturally, and for your cardio workouts I suggest the Full-Body Swimming Toning Workout on page 150.

10 BUST-TONING MOVES

Each exercise has a suggested number of repetitions (e.g., the amount of times you perform the exercise) as well as how many sets you do. As you become fitter each week, you can adapt the workout. For example, for the first week do the recommended amounts for a beginner, then progress to intermediate the next week, and then to advanced the final week.

Additionally, the stars next to each exercise allow you to grade how hard the exercise is:

✳   Light

✳✳   Moderate

✳✳✳   Hard

7

Bust Press ✻

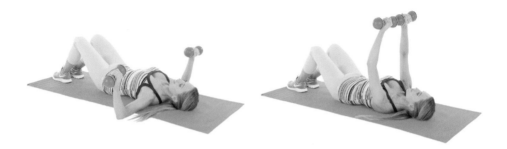

Step 1: Lie face up on your mat with your knees bent and feet firmly on the floor. Your arms are out to your side, with your elbows bent, and holding on to your weights with your palms facing away from the body.

Step 2: Slowly extend your arms straight up, keeping them in line with the bust. Hold for a second, and then slowly lower the arms down. Be sure to keep your tummy muscles pulled in as you lift and lower your arms.

Beginner: 12-14 reps, 2 sets
Intermediate: 16-18 reps, 3 sets
Advanced: 20 reps, 4 sets

Killer Cleavage Lift ★★

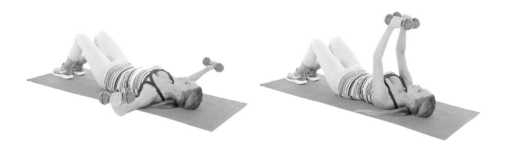

Step 1: Lie face up on your mat with your knees bent and feet firmly on the floor. Take your arms out wide to your sides, palms facing up. Slightly bend the arms.

Step 2: Pull in your tummy muscles while simultaneously drawing both your arms up until they meet in the middle above the head, keeping them in line with your bust. Hold, and then slowly lower back down to the starting position.

Beginner:	8-10 reps, 2 sets
Intermediate:	12-14 reps, 3 sets
Advanced:	20 reps, 3 sets

7

Wonder Bust Press ✱✱

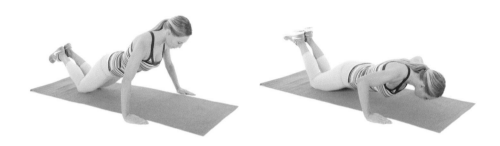

Step 1: Kneel on your mat, with your hands wider than shoulder-width distance apart and in line with your shoulders. Gently come onto the fleshy part of your knees and push your hips forward. You are trying for a straight line from your knees to your head.

Step 2: Slowly lower your upper body down towards the ground by bending through your elbows and letting them flare out to the side. Keep your abs pulled in at the same time. Hold, and then slowly push back up to the starting position.

Beginner: 6-8 reps, 2 sets
Intermediate: 10-12 reps, 3 sets
Advanced: 20 reps, 3 sets

Book Bust Toner ✿✿

Step 1: Using a book, come into a fully extended plank position with both hands firmly placed on the book (the bigger the book, the harder the work).

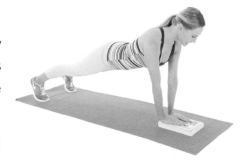

Step 2: Walk one hand off the book, hold and then walk the same hand back on. Then walk the opposite hand off the book, and walk it back on again. Keep repeating this for the required reps. Be sure to keep your tummy muscles fully engaged throughout the exercise.

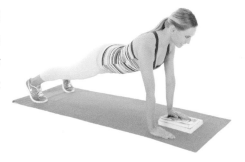

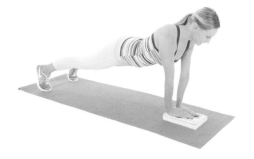

Beginner:	10 reps, 2 sets
Intermediate:	16 reps, 3 sets
Advanced:	20 reps, 4 sets

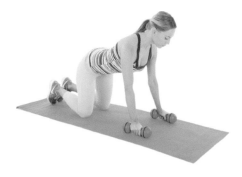

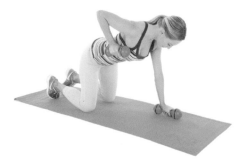

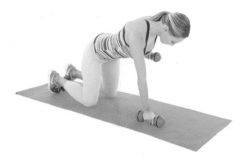

Bra Enhancer ⭐

Step 1: Kneeling on all fours, hold on to your hand weights. Fully engage your core muscles by pulling in your tummy tight.

Step 2: Ease one arm up by bending through your elbow, aiming to get the weight by your shoulder. Hold for a second, and then slowly lower. Alternate from side to side for the required reps. It is important to keep your hips still as you do this, so be sure to keep the tummy pulled in.

Beginner: 14 reps, 2 sets
Intermediate: 16 reps, 3 sets
Advanced: 20 reps, 4 sets

Power Push ★★★

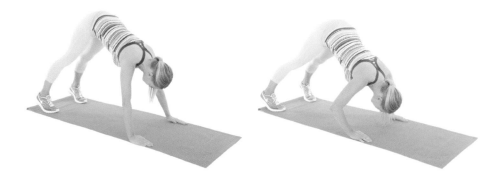

Step 1: Get onto all fours and form a V shape. Your hands should be shoulder-width distance apart and slightly in front of your shoulders. Lift your heels off the ground.

Step 2: Very slowly bend through your elbows slightly so that you are lowering your head down towards the ground. Only lower a couple of inches, and then push back up. Keep repeating this for the required reps. It is important to slowly come down into a sitting position after this for a few seconds, and do not jump straight back up to standing or you'll experience a head rush.

7

Beginner:	6 reps, 2 sets
Intermediate:	10 reps, 3 sets
Advanced:	14 reps, 4 sets

Book Press ⭐

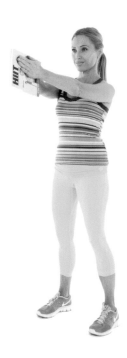 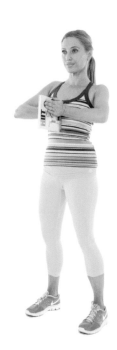

Step 1: Stand with your feet hip-width distance apart, with your knees slightly bent. Hold a book between your palms. Your fingers should be pointing forwards and your arms fully extended at chest height, squeezing as tightly as you can.

Step 2: Maintaining the squeeze, draw the book towards the centre of your chest, bending your elbows out the side. The important part of this exercise is to maintain that squeeze. Then return to the starting position.

Beginner: 16 reps, 2 sets

Intermediate: 20 reps, 3 sets

Advanced: 30 reps, 4 sets

Towel Squeeze ✴

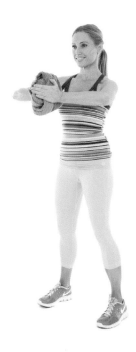 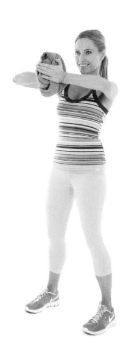

7

Step 1: Holding a towel between your palms, stand with your feet slightly wider than hip-width distance apart, your knees slightly bent and your tummy muscles pulled in. Your elbows should be bent and in line with your bust.

Step 2: Now try to squeeze the towel as hard as you can. Imagine you are trying to get any excess water out. Hold the squeeze, and then lift the towel a couple of inches directly upwards. Hold, and then lower back to your starting position, still squeezing hard. Repeat.

Beginner:	12 reps, 2 sets
Intermediate:	16 reps, 3 sets
Advanced:	20 reps, 4 sets

L Shape Bust Lift ★★

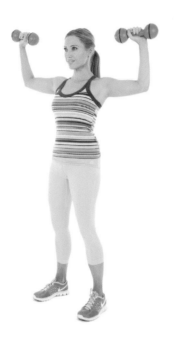 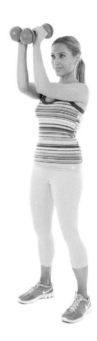

Step 1: Stand with good posture and tummy pulled in. Hold on to your hand weights with both palms facing in, arms out to each side and elbows bent so that your arms form an L shape, with your elbows in line with your shoulders.

Step 2: Keeping the arms at the same height, slowly bring them together so that your forearms meet in the middle. Hold, then take back out to the starting position.

Beginner: 8-10 reps, 2 sets
Intermediate: 14-16 reps, 3 sets
Advanced: 20 reps, 4 sets

Natural Bust Lift ★★

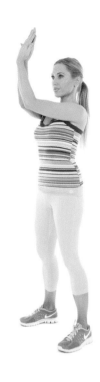 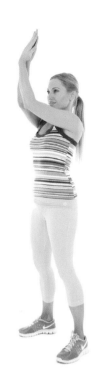

Step 1: Stand with your feet slightly wider than hip-width distance apart, your knees slightly bent and your tummy muscles pulled in. Bend your arms in front of you, with one hand crossed over the other.

Step 2: Maintaining the same arm position, ease your arms several inches higher. Hold, and then lower back to the starting position.

Beginner:	20 reps, 2 sets
Intermediate:	30 reps, 3 sets
Advanced:	50 reps, 4 sets

FREQUENTLY ASKED QUESTIONS: BUST

Question: My bust has started to sag after having children; is there anything I can do about this?

Answer: Yes, as I mention in the beginning of this chapter, we can naturally lift our bust by targeting the Cooper's ligament – this is the equivalent of a human bra strap. The tighter this is, the more lifted your bust becomes, so by activating this muscle we can lift the bust.

Question: Is it important to wear a sports bra when you are working out?

Answer: 100 per cent YES as your breasts move from side to side and up and down as you move, and without full support this can damage your connective muscles tissue. And don't think that is only for the bigger busts. It is important for even for the more petite. So you can still do you workouts in your PJs! Just make sure you always have on your sports bra and your trainers.

MEASURE YOUR PROGRESS

Bust fitness

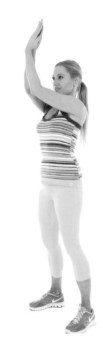

To measure and see how much you have improved your muscular strength and endurance through your bust, I recommend that you do the Natural Bust Lift every couple of weeks. Perform as many as you can, and keep a note of your score. Every couple of weeks you will see that you can perform more.

You will start to notice that your bust lifts as the muscles start to tone up. Measure this by using a tape measure. You can choose either left or right, but be sure to always do the same side each time you measure. Start at the top of your shoulder and let the tape measure hang down vertically to your nipple line. Make a note of this measurement, and then measure this every couple of weeks. Be sure to do it in the same spot.

BUST BEAUTY TIP

A great way to firm and smooth out the skin on your bust is by doing this DIY bust veil mask of mine. This only requires three natural ingredients and just one other thing – an old bra!

Ingredients:
1 tablespoon of natural yoghurt
½ teaspoon of oatmeal
1 teaspoon of vitamin E oil

Mix all the ingredients together thoroughly. Apply this mixture over the bust and then put on the old bra. Leave this mixture on for 15 minutes. This allows the skin to absorb the nutrients. After 15 minutes, remove the mixture by rinsing off with cold water. And this combined with your toning exercises from my book will give you that wonder bust.

8 ARMS

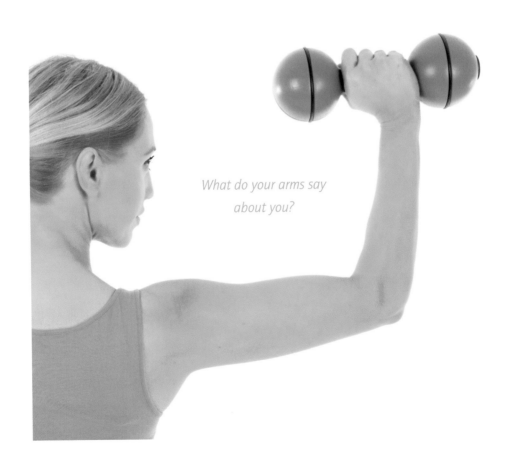

*What do your arms say
about you?*

Your arms can be a giveaway to your lifestyle and habits, as you can see if an individual is fit and healthy by her arms! Are they toned and strong, or are they saggy and baggy? The saggy and baggy arms indicate being unfit, not taking regular exercise and eating a high calorie diet, whereas the toned and lean arms indicate a healthy diet and active lifestyle.

Our arms are in use from the minute we wake to the last thing at night, from brushing our teeth to carrying shopping bags, so even within our daily chores we use and engage our arms. The arms especially engaged in certain exercises, such as running in which it is your arms that help to propel you forwards. Yet even though we use our arms pretty much non-stop, we can still have toned arms, as the secret to beautifully sculpted and toned arms is toning all the various arm muscles and tightening and sculpting from every angle.

The arms, just like our butt and abs, can easily store body fat and lose their tone. Yet with the right exercises and workout plan we can have the arms we have dreamed of and say goodbye to what are often referred to as Bingo Wings, Auntie's Arms and Bat Wings.

And this is good, as the arms tend to be more on show than other areas, especially in the warmer months when we can live in t-shirts, tank tops and sleeveless dresses.

As a fitness expert, I can tell you that toning, strengthening and sculpting your arms is actually quite easy. And with a combination of strength training moves and cardio

8

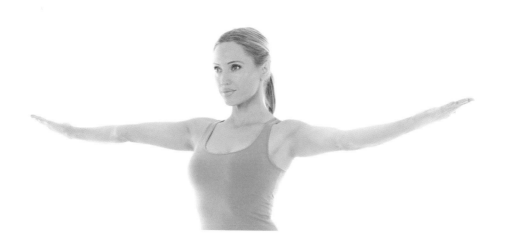

exercise we are going to reduce your overall excess body fat. Some people find that when they start to lose weight it comes off their butt, or their abs, and others their arms. The good news is that when we reach a healthy body weight, we then have less excess body fat overall. All my toning moves that are specific to the arms mean that you can find your beautifully sculpted arms.

Women tend to notice that they lose the tone in the back of the upper arm. This is known as the *triceps* muscle, which runs down the back of the upper arm and is attached from the back of your shoulder to the elbow. This gets less challenged than the muscles at the front of our arm, known as the *biceps* (think of them as neighbours). This muscle is attached from the front of your shoulder to the front of your elbow, but we naturally engage this muscle a lot more, for example, carrying shopping bags and lifting up items, and so it tends to stay more toned. The shoulders have the muscles known as the *deltoids*, and the stronger and better toned these are, the more they showcase sexy shoulders and also help improve posture so that you have an elegant shape. And better upper-body posture can instantly make us look slimmer and like we are oozing with confidence.

These exercises will help you achieve the toned arms that will give you the freedom to ditch cardigans and go sleeveless.

THE BENEFITS OF TONING THIS AREA

- You will look more feminine.

- You will feel that you have more strength in your arms and upper body.

- You will have sexy, sculpted shoulders.

- You will lose excess arm fat.

- You will tone and tighten your arms.

- You will be happy to wave your arms.

- You will feel confident to go sleeveless.

○ You will have better upper-body flexibility.

○ You will burn more calories as you become more toned.

○ You will have better posture.

So let's get those arms t-shirt friendly.

I have created and put together 10 different strength training exercises for your arms, so you will have plenty of variations and never get bored. We are also going to look at cardio. Powerwalking, like in the 16-Minute Fat-Burning Powerwalk (page 149), is a great way to help shift any excess body fat.

10 LEG-TONING MOVES

Each exercise has a suggested number of repetitions (e.g., the amount of times you perform the exercise) as well as how many sets you do. As you become fitter each week, you can adapt the workout. For example, for the first week do the recommended amounts for a beginner, then progress to intermediate the next week, and then to advanced the final week.

Additionally, the stars next to each exercise allow you to grade how hard the exercise is:

⭐ Light

⭐⭐ Moderate

⭐⭐⭐ Hard

Banish Bingo Wing Squeeze ⭐

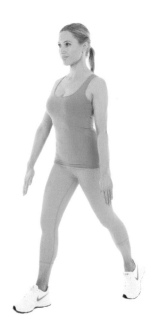
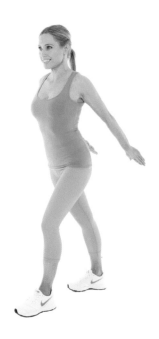

Step 1: Start in a split stance, with tummy pulled in, chest lifted, arms straight down by your sides and your palms facing directly behind you.

Step 2: Now lift your arms straight out directly behind you, lifting them as high as you can, and hold. Then perform tiny little pulses. It is important that you keep the arms at the same height. Aim to do 100 of these. Halfway through change your stance so that the opposite leg is in front.

Beginner: 50 reps, 1 sets
Intermediate: 50 reps, 2 sets
Advanced: 100 reps, 2 sets

Sexy Shoulder Sculptor ✳

Step 1: Stand in a split stance, with your knees slightly bent, tummy pulled in and your arms slightly bent and out to your sides, palms facing up.

Step 2: Slowly draw both your arms to the centre, crossing one over the other. Hold, still keeping your palms facing up, then slowly open back out to starting position. Then cross over again, with the other arm crossing over the top. Repeat for the required reps.

Beginner: 20 reps, 2 sets
Intermediate: 30 reps, 3 sets
Advanced: 50 reps, 3 sets

A-Lister Arms ★★

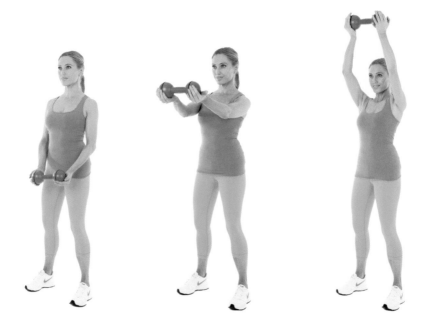

Step 1: Stand with good posture and your knees slightly bent and tummy pulled in. Hold on to your weight with an underhand grip (palms are facing up). Your hands should be shoulder-width distance apart.

Step 2: Slowly start to raise your arms up until they are directly above you, keeping your tummy muscles pulled in tight to protect your back. Hold for a second, and then slowly lower back to the starting position.

Beginner: 8 reps, 2 sets
Intermediate: 12-14 reps, 3 sets
Advanced: 25 reps, 3 sets

Arm-Boosting Lift ★★

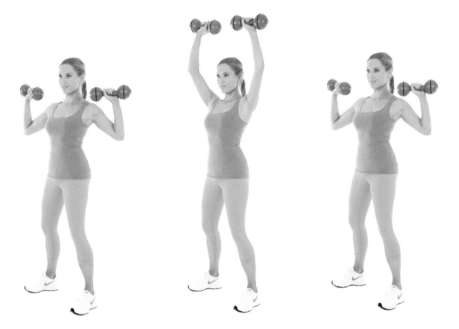

Step 1: Stand with your feet hip-width distance apart and your knees slightly bent, tummy pulled in. Hold on to your weights, with your palms facing forwards and your elbows bent out to your sides.

Step 2: In a controlled manner lift both arms directly above your head, hold, and then slowly lower back to your starting position.

Beginner: 10-12 reps, 2 sets
Intermediate: 14-16 reps, 3 sets
Advanced: 20 reps, 3 sets

V Lift ★★

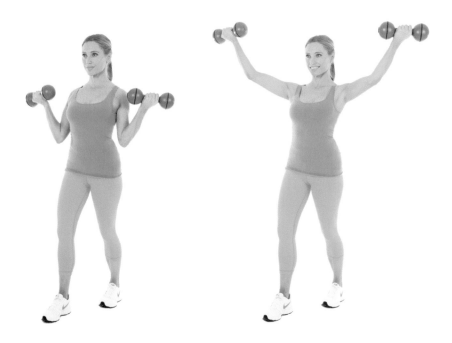

Step 1: Stand in a split stance with good posture and your abdominals engaged. Pull your elbows close into your sides and hold on to your weights, with your palms facing behind you.

Step 2: Now slowly lift your arms up and out so you create a V shape, still keeping a slight bend in the arms. Hold, and then slowly lower back to the starting position.

Beginner: 8-10 reps, 2 sets
Intermediate: 12-14 reps, 3 sets
Advanced: 16-18 reps, 3 sets

Arm Circles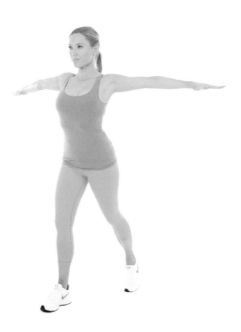

Step 1: Stand in a split stance with feet hip-width distance apart and arms out to your sides so that your body forms a T shape.

Step 2: Start slowly making small circular motions with your arms in a clockwise direction. Then make small circular motions in a counterclockwise direction for the required reps.

8

Beginner: 30 reps one direction, then 30 reps the other direction, 2 sets

Intermediate: 40 reps one direction, then 50 reps the other direction, 2 sets

Advanced: 50 reps one direction, then 50 reps the other direction, 2 sets

Go Sleeveless Arm Curl ✲

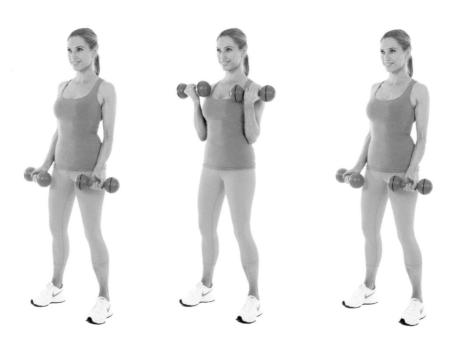

Step 1: Stand with your feet hip-width distance apart and your knees slightly bent and tummy pulled in. Arms are down by your side, holding on to your weights with an overhand grip, meaning your palms are facing up.

Step 2: Now gently lift the weights up to your shoulders while still keeping your elbows in the same position, hold and then slowly lower back to your starting position.

Beginner: 10 reps, 2 sets
Intermediate: 12-14 reps, 3 sets
Advanced: 20 reps, 3 sets

Goodbye Baggy Arms ✲✲✲

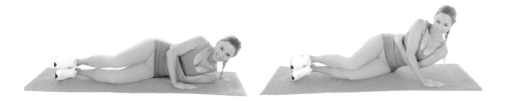

Step 1: Lying on your mat on your side with your knees slightly bent, wrap your bottom arm around your ribcage, and place your top arm firmly on the ground in front of you in line with your chest.

Step 2: Now press through the palm of the hand on the floor and slightly lift your upper body off the floor, coming up as high as you can. Hold, and then slowly lower back down.

Beginner: 6 reps, 2 sets
Intermediate: 8-10 reps, 3 sets
Advanced: 15 reps, 3 sets

8

Love Your Arms Press ★★✿

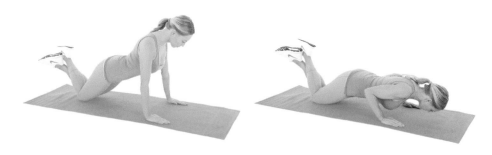

Step 1: Kneel on a mat with your hips pressed forwards and tummy pulled in. Your hands are directly under your shoulders with your fingers pointing forwards.

Step 2: In a controlled manner, lower your upper body down to the ground, making sure you keep your elbows tight to your sides and don't let them flare out. Hold, and then slowly push back up.

Beginner: 6 reps, 2 sets
Intermediate: 10 reps, 3 sets
Advanced: 15 reps, 3 sets

Dip for Delicious Arms ✦

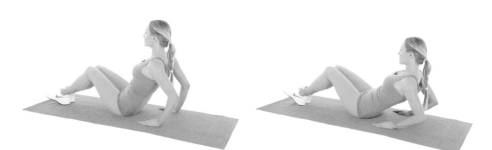

Step 1: Sit on the ground with your knees bent and your hands behind you (about six inches away), with fingertips pointing forwards and elbows pointing directly backwards.

Step 2: Now gently lower back by bending through your elbows, making sure you keep the elbows tucked in. Hold, and then slowly push back up to the starting position.

8

Beginner: 10 reps, 2 sets
Intermediate: 14-16 reps, 3 sets
Advanced: 20 reps, 3 sets

FREQUENTLY ASKED QUESTIONS: ARMS

Question: As I get older the back of my arms are getting fatter and less toned. Is there anything I can do?

Answer: Yes, this sort of change generally happens as we age, and if we do not alter our lifestyle habits then it can take its toll on our body, often the arms first. But the good news is that with healthy and active living you can reverse this and get back those toned slim arms.

Question: What is the best cardio exercise to do that will also help tone my arms?

Answer: There are two exercises that win, hands down. The first is swimming, as your arms are big players in the water. Swimming will work all your arm muscles, and in different ways, when you do a mix of strokes – from front crawl to breaststroke to backstroke. And then the second great cardio workout is walking, and even more so if you have a couple of light hand weights you can carry while you walk; then when you swing the arms as you walk you will also be toning.

Question: Will lifting weights give me big bulky arms?

Answer: Not in the way that we do the exercises in this book, and to be honest you would have to train in a very specific manner to develop big bulky arms. In this book we use smaller weights, and for a lot of the exercise we are simply using our own body weight. So the answer is that by lifting small weights and using your own body weight you won't get bulky arms, but rather lean sculpted arms.

MEASURE YOUR PROGRESS

Arm fitness

It's good to measure and see how much you have improved your muscular strength and endurance through your arms with time. I recommend that you do this by performing the Love Your Arms Press every couple of weeks. Perform as many as you can and keep a note of your score, as every couple of weeks you should find you can perform more.

You will start to notice that
your arms change shape as
the inches come down and
the muscles start to tone
up, and this can also be
measured.

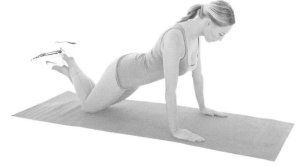

Using your right arm, place
a tape measure around the
upper arm approximately a hand's distance from your shoulder, and note the measurement.
Then measure this every couple of weeks, being sure to do it in the same spot.

ARM BEAUTY TIP

8

So now that you have worked hard on shaping and toning your arms and you are ready to
throw off that cardigan and display your sleek arms, try this DIY silky smooth arm scrub
of mine.

Ingredients:
Virgin olive oil
Sugar
Drop of lavender oil

In a small bowl pour in a tablespoon of olive oil then a teaspoon of sugar and a few drops
of lavender oil. Mix together, and then apply this in the bath. Start at your hands and rub
all the way up to the top of your arms, leave on for 10 minutes, and then gently wash off
and pat dry.

This will leave you with the silkiest, smoothest skin, and you will now love your arms even
more.

9 BACK

A strong back is a quick way to look years younger.

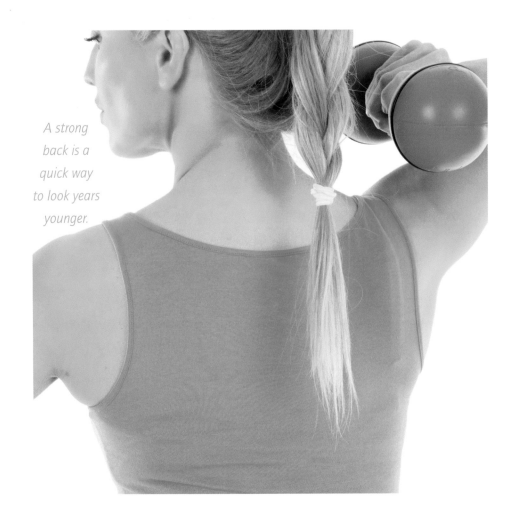

Our backs are often overused, neglected and put under a lot of pressure when long hours are spent working on computers. Even simple things such as driving can play havoc with your back. This is why this area is so important to keep toned and strong so that no matter how long we spend in front of the computer, we can still have a well-maintained back.

A strong back not only gives you elegant and perfect posture, but it will also make you look leaner and taller. And remember that the more toned our muscles, the more calories we burn, so doing your back exercises will not only help sculpt you a beautiful back, but it will also help increase your calorie burn!

The back has lots of big muscle groups, such as the *trapezius*, located on the upper back, as well as the *deltoids* and *rhomboids*, and in the middle of your back you have a big muscle known as the *latissimus dorsi*. Then another important muscle in your back is known as the *erector spinae*, and this runs down either side of your spine. Keeping these toned and strong will not only protect your spine, but it will also have the extra benefit of improving your balance and flexibility. And also the more toned your back is, the more lifted your chest is, which in turn helps lift your bust, helping create a feminine shape.

9

THE BENEFITS OF TONING THIS AREA

○ You will have better posture.

○ You will have a stronger back.

○ You will increase your calorie burn.

○ You will smooth out any back fat.

○ You will look super confident.

For the cardio exercise I recommend swimming, as this is one of the best ways to strengthen, tone and sculpt your back and your core, and it also engages your butt and lower leg muscles. See page 150 for the Full-Body Swimming Toning Workout

10 BACK-TONING MOVES

Each exercise has a suggested number of repetitions (e.g., the amount of times you perform the exercise) as well as how many sets you do. As you become fitter each week, you can adapt the workout. For example, for the first week do the recommended amounts for a beginner, then progress to intermediate the next week, and then to advanced the final week.

Additionally, the stars next to each exercise allow you to grade how hard the exercise is:

⭐ Light

⭐⭐ Moderate

⭐⭐⭐ Hard

9

Back Lift ★★

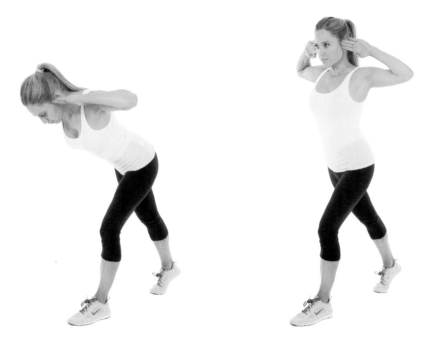

Step 1: Stand in a split stance with your feet hip-width distance apart and your arms bent with fingertips by the side of your head. Tilt forward from your hips, being sure to keep your tummy pulled in tight.

Step 2: Focusing on using your abdominal muscles, lift your upper body to a straight position. Hold, and then slowly lower back to your starting position. Keep repeating. Always keep the tummy pulled in.

Beginner:	8 reps, 2 sets
Intermediate:	10 reps, 3 sets
Advanced:	14 reps, 3 sets

Spreading Wings Lift ⭐⭐

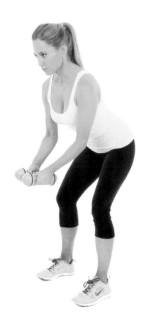 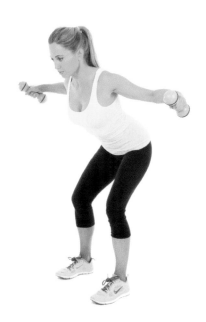

9

Step 1: Stand with your knees slightly bent and feet hip-width distance apart, leaning slightly forwards. Hold on to your weights, which you should place together in front of you. Keep your abdominals pulled in.

Step 2: Now lift both arms out to your sides, and imagine you are trying to squeeze your shoulder blades together. Still keep a slight bend in the elbows. Hold, and then lower back to your starting position.

Beginner:	8 reps, 2 sets
Intermediate:	10 reps, 3 sets
Advanced:	16 reps, 3 sets

Goodbye to Back Fat Lift ⭐

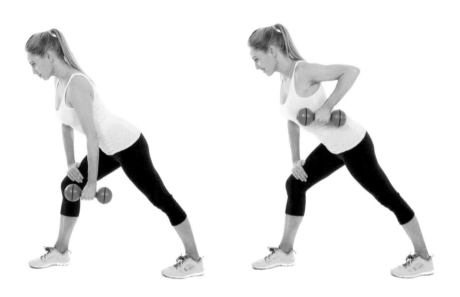

Step 1: Stand in a deep split stance with a hand on the bent leg and the opposite leg fully extended back. The other arm hangs down and holds on to the weight with your palm facing in.

Step 2: In a controlled manner, bend the extended arm and lift the weight up towards your shoulder. Hold for a second, and then slowly lower. Repeat on the same arm for the required reps before switching arms.

Beginner: 10 reps, 3 sets
Intermediate: 12-14 reps, 3 sets
Advanced: 20 reps, 3 sets

Bow and Arrow ✿✿

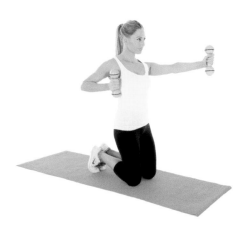

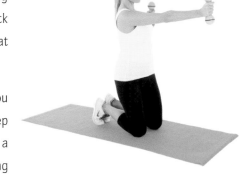

9

Step 1: Kneel on your mat and hold on to your weights, with your palms facing inwards. Start with one arm pulled back and the other extended forwards, both at shoulder height.

Step 2: Now change arms, and imagine you are using a bow and arrow. Be sure to keep your tummy muscles pulled in. Hold for a second or two, and then return to starting position. If you find kneeling uncomfortable, you can also perform this standing up.

Beginner:	14 reps, 2 sets
Intermediate:	18 reps, 2 sets
Advanced:	20 reps, 3 sets

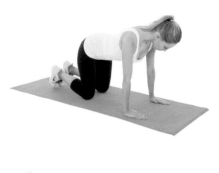

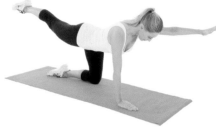

Superwoman ✿✿

Step 1: Kneel on the mat on all fours, making sure your hands are directly under your shoulders and knees are under your hips.

Step 2: Making sure to keep your hips still by pulling your tummy muscles in and up, hold, and then slowly extend one arm and the opposite leg simultaneously so that you form a straight line. Hold, and then slowly lower to your starting position. Alternate sides for the required reps.

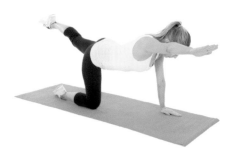

Beginner:	8 reps, 2 sets
Intermediate:	10 reps, 3 sets
Advanced:	20 reps, 3 sets

Posture Perfect Lift ✿✿

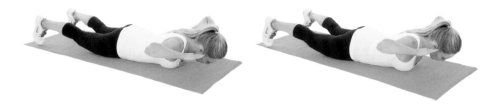

Step 1: Lie facedown on your mat, with arms bent and out to your sides and your fingertips by your ears.

Step 2: Very slowly lift your head and shoulders up (not too high). Hold, and then slowly lower back to your starting position. This is a small move; focus on doing it slowly.

Beginner:	10 reps, 2 sets
Intermediate:	12 reps, 3 sets
Advanced:	20 reps, 3 sets

Swim It Off ✿✿

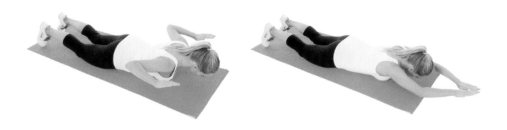

Step 1: Lie facedown on your mat, with your head and chest slightly lifted off the ground and your arms bent at your sides, palms facing down.

Step 2: Still keeping your head and chest lifted, extend the arms directly forward, as if you are swimming. Then bring them back to your starting position. Keep repeating.

Beginner:	8 reps, 2 sets
Intermediate:	10 reps, 3 sets
Advanced:	20 reps, 3 sets

Back Sculptor ✹✹✹

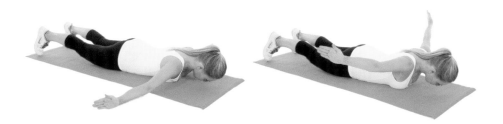

Step 1: Lie facedown on your mat and extend both arms out to either side, keeping your hands in line with your shoulders, with your palms facing forwards and thumbs pointing up to the ceiling.

Step 2: Now lift both arms up high and out to your sides by squeezing your shoulder blades together. Hold, and then slowly lower back to your starting position.

Beginner:	6 reps, 2 sets
Intermediate:	10 reps, 3 sets
Advanced:	16 reps, 3 sets

Banish the Bra Bulge ★★

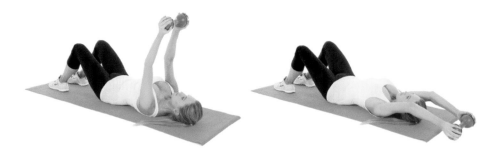

Step 1: Lie face up, with your knees bent and feet flat on the floor. Hold on to your weight with your arms directly above you. Pull in your tummy muscles.

Step 2: Now slowly lower the weight down towards the ground. Hold, and then gently draw back up to the starting position. At all times keep the tummy muscles pulled in.

Beginner: 8 reps, 2 sets
Intermediate: 10 reps, 3 sets
Advanced: 16 reps, 3 sets

Back Arm Walk ⭐⭐

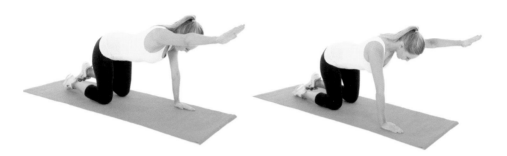

Step 1: Kneel on your mat, with your hips directly over your knees and one arm directly straight out in front of you, the other firmly placed on the floor.

Step 2: Now bring the straight arm down to the floor and lift the opposite arm, at all times keeping the tummy pulled in. Alternate from arm to arm for the required reps.

Beginner:	10 reps, 2 sets
Intermediate:	14 reps, 3 sets
Advanced:	20 reps, 3 sets

9

FREQUENTLY ASKED QUESTIONS: BACK

Question: Is there any way I can get rid of the back fat that causes an overhang around my bra line?

Answer: Yes. Our back, just like any part of our body, can store excess body fat, but by doing a combination of cardio exercise, as I suggest in this book, and doing the back strengthening and toning exercises, you will notice those bulges dramatically start to disappear.

Question: I play tennis. Are there any good back exercises I can do to help improve my swing?

Answer: Yes. A great one that you could do would be the Back Sculptor. Not only does that engage your latissimus dorsi muscle, which facilitates your swing, but this one also helps increase your chest flexibility, ensuring you will then have a great range of motion in your swing—and more power to it, too.

Question: I had a back injury a while ago, so I don't like to do any high-impact aerobic exercise. What would you recommend I do that will be gentle on my back?

Answer: Walking would be a good choice, as this is lower impact. And you can focus on doing it with good posture. I would recommend you do it on an even surface and avoid any cross-country, as uneven ground can be uncomfortable on your joints and have a knock-on effect on your back. Other exercises that are back friendly are swimming and even gentle rowing, as long as you are doing it with good form.

MEASURE YOUR PROGRESS

Back fitness

Each week you will find that the back becomes stronger, and you are able to perform more repetitions of each move. To measure your back strength, see how many Perfect Posture Lifts you can perform before your back starts to feel challenged. Make a note of this and then do the measurement every two weeks.

Back measurements

The back muscles will tone quickly when doing these workouts, and you will notice some exciting results, especially if you are focusing on eating a healthy diet and doing some cardio 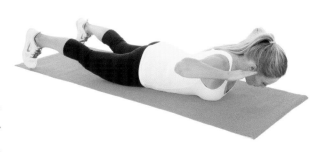 workouts. Using a tape measure, measure your back by placing the tape measure about 1 inch below your armpit and wrapping it around you horizontally. Make a note of your measurement and then do this every two weeks.

9

BACK BEAUTY TIP

So let's be honest, this one is going to be a pretty hard area to apply one of my homemade lotions to, so instead we are going to look at a great tip on how we can keep your back looking beautiful.

You will need some small stickers to serve as simple visual reminders for you. I would like you to stick them on your steering wheel if you drive, on your computer, on your bathroom mirror or even on the television. They can be small, but every time you see this sticker I want you to instantly alter your posture so that it is perfect. And a great way of doing this is to imagine that someone has dropped an ice cube down your back, and you will instantly pull those shoulders back. The more time we spend having good posture, the more we automatically retain better posture.

10 CARDIO

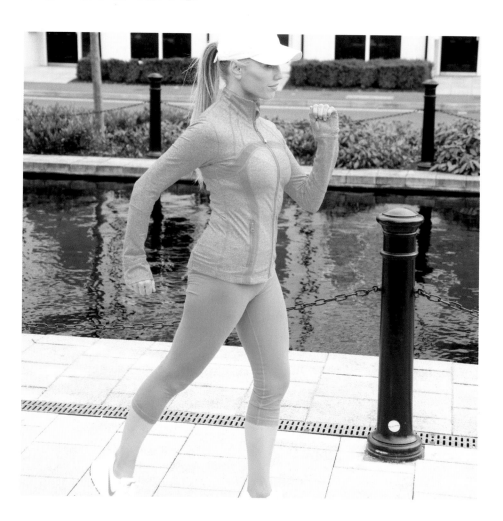

As your trainer the most important thing I want to provide for you in all my workouts, apps, and books is RESULTS, and adding in cardio is going to speed up your results. And if you have any excess body fat, this will help melt it off, so you will be able to see the underlying muscles that you have toned and sculpted from the exercises in my book.

Cardio exercise is different from strength training and toning. Cardio, also known as aerobic exercise, simply gets your heart beating faster than usual for a set period of time, which helps to keep the heart and lungs healthy, reduces blood pressure, lowers stress levels and helps keep us fit and positive. And one extra benefit of cardio exercise that tends to motivate most women is that by working out we increase the levels of the *human growth hormone*, which is the hormone that is responsible for keeping our skin plumped up, with that youthful glow, so think of exercise as the best anti-aging treatment money can buy!

10

I have created four different cardio workouts, with suggestions as to which areas for the body they particularly complement. All have amazing effects on overall tone, so you can pick and choose or simply try whatever takes your fancy on the day.

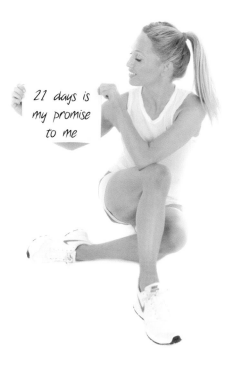

21 days is my promise to me

It is important to always warm up first before you exercise and perform all the stretches which are on pages 32-34, and then at the end of the workout cool down and stretch.

I recommend you do cardio training three times a week, as this way you will be well on track to reach those dream goals within 21 days.

POWERWALKING WORKOUT

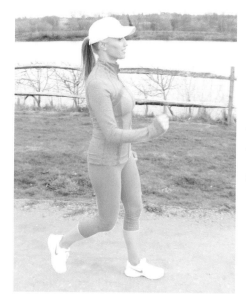

Powerwalking is one of my personal favourite cardio exercises, as it is low impact but can get great results. Powerwalking is simply walking a little faster than normal, and this move means as you are walking faster you naturally engage your arms more. You can also use your small hand weights and tone your arms at the same time.

Technique

- Ensure you walk with good posture.

- Keep your tummy muscles pulled in.

- Keep your hips facing forwards as you walk.

- Aim as you walk to land your heel first and then roll off from your toes.

- Always do your warm-up and stretches.

16-MINUTE FAT-BURNING POWERWALK

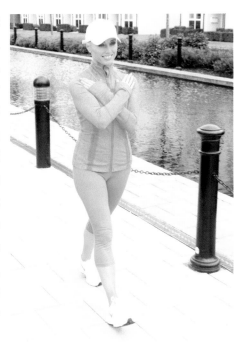

We are going to focus on three different strides which will all target a certain area. The first will simply be your **Powerwalking**. Then the second is focusing more on your butt and thighs by doing the **Butt and Thigh Stride**. You do this by powerwalking at your brisk pace with your arms crossed and resting on your chest (this means you work the lower body harder, as all the effort comes from the legs, whereas normally the arms, as they swing back and forth, help to propel your faster). You can feel the bottom, abs and thighs working harder. Still focus on keeping good posture, making sure your shoulders stay in line with your hips.

10

And then the third stride is the **Arm Sculptor**. You do this by powerwalking at your brisk pace but now really focusing on pumping through with your arms. The faster you pump your arms, the faster you walk, so you will instantly find that you are walking faster, while you will find your stride will shorten slightly as you pick up your pace.

16-Minute Fat-Burning Powerwalk

2 minutes	Powerwalk at a brisk pace
1 minute	Butt and thigh stride
1 minute	Arm sculptor stride

Repeat this sequence a total of 4 times.

SWIMMING WORKOUT

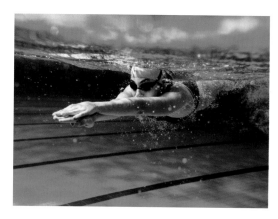

Swimming is a great way to tone all over without putting any impact on your joints, and this water workout will suit every fitness level and will help reduce body fat. I have designed this workout to give you a full-body toning workout, but you only need to stick to a 20-minute swim and can use your favourite strokes.

Technique

○ Always perform each move and stroke with good form.

○ Always warm up and cool down before and after the workout.

Full-Body Swimming Toning Workout

○ Start off in the shallow end so that the water is at your chest height. Do 6 laps of walking from one side to the other, just doing widths.

○ Now swim 6 lengths of the pool (ideally front crawl).

○ Then walk 4 widths of the shallow end.

○ Next swim 4 lengths (ideally breaststroke).

○ Walk 2 widths.

○ Then finish off swimming 2 lengths (ideally backstroke).

Note: You can perform the stroke that you feel most comfortable with. These here are only suggestions, so please feel free to stick with your usual swimming style.

RUNNING WORKOUT

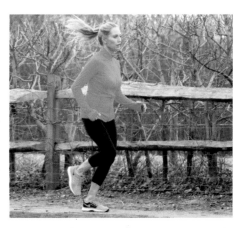

Running is a great cardiovascular workout, and it can burn off calories fast. It is also a great way to work off stress. Running will tone you all over and is a sure way to help reduce any excess tummy fat. You can stick with your normal run or try this high-intensity interval running plan of mine taken from my book, *HIIT*. This works on shorter periods where you up the speed of your run to a faster pace, and it is these little short bursts of high intensity that help speed up your calorie burn and fitness levels.

10

Technique

- Always run with good form.

- Aim to keep your chest open and shoulders pulled back.

- Avoid overly clenching your fists, and aim to land softly.

- Always warm up and cool down.

15-Minute HIIT Run

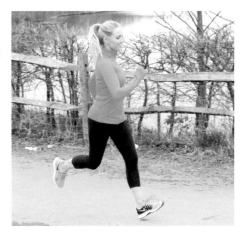

- 2 minutes and 30 seconds running at a normal pace.

- 20 seconds sprinting as fast as you can.

- 10 seconds gentle jog.

- Repeat this sequence 5 times in total.

STEPS WORKOUT

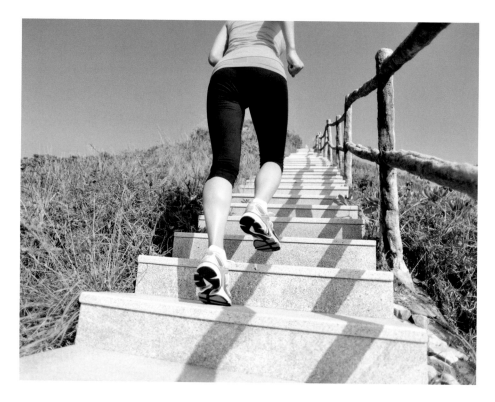

Steps or stairs are great for lifting and sculpting your butt, and you can either do this at home or head outdoors to find some good steps. This will get your heart rate up, so you get a great cardio workout at the same time.

Technique

○ Always make sure your feet are firmly on the step.

○ Avoid using any steps that have a slippery surface or are unsecure.

○ Always aim to step with good posture.

○ Always warm up and cool down before and after the workout.

○ Aim to find a set of steps/stairs that have at least 10.

10 STEPS TO PERFECT TONE WORKOUT

1. Standing at base of stairs, run up to tenth step, and then slowly walk back down.

2. At the base of the steps perform 10 squats; see page 65.

3. Run up to the eighth step, and then slowly march back down.

4. At the base of the steps perform 8 squats.

5. Run up to the sixth step, and then slowly march back down.

6. At the base of the steps perform 6 squats.

7. Run up to the fourth step, and then slowly march back down.

8. At the base of the steps perform 4 squats.

9. Run up to the second step, and then slowly march back down.

10. At the base of the steps perform 2 squats.

10

Part 3

11 DIET

Food is to be enjoyed, and eating the right foods in your diet is just like going to a health spa, as you are pampering your body from the inside out.

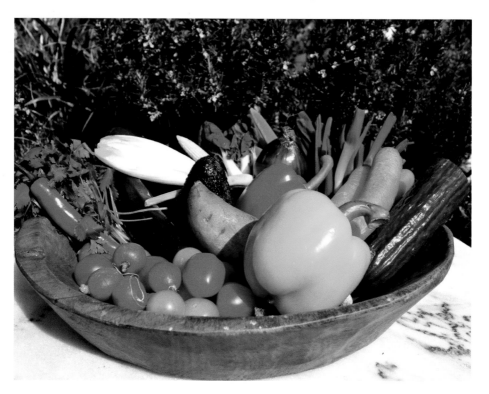

WHAT IS A HEALTHY CLEAN DIET?

So just what is a clean and healthy diet? Well by this I mean we simply avoid any processed foods and have a diet that is natural as nature intended and not stuffed full of chemicals and preservatives, which at the end of the day are just being used by the manufacturers to make themselves a fat profit at the risk of your health. These foods are designed to look appealing, to have a longer shelf life and to get your taste buds hooked, but would we really be that tempted to eat those processed foods, meals, snacks, drinks or cereals if we knew the damage that they can do to our insides and the effects they can have on our weight, health and energy, and how quickly we age?

The good news is that on a healthy clean diet you can still have as many mouth-watering favourite meals, snacks or treats as you desire.

There is nothing quite like home cooking, and I have wonderful memories of the tasty treats my mum would prepare for me and my sister when we were growing up. We lived way out in the countryside, and my mum would utilise all the foods that we grew there. Being an amazing artist, her creativity always shines through in whatever she does, and not only did the food taste delicious, but it also looked really vibrant and appealing. My sister has carried on this family skill and is an incredible cook, who, with four beautiful children with a variety of food allergies, has continued this practice of creating healthy home-cooked meals, which can do us nothing but good.

With this chapter I wanted to show you some of my favourite simple dishes that are easy to create, are stuffed full of goodness and look as good as they taste. And the final benefit is that every single one of these delicious dishes will nourish your body to the maximum.

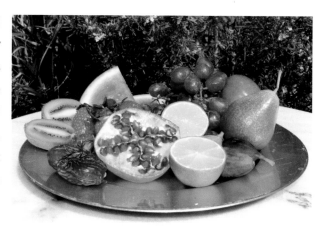

RECIPES

Let's start with my favourite decadent-feeling breakfast.

Super antioxidant breakfast

Chia-seed raspberry jam with figs and crunchy apple and cinnamon dip washed down with a Lime Detox Fizz—this really is one of the purest and healthiest breakfasts you can kick-start your day with.

Here's why this breakfast is one of the best and could easily win first place in the healthiest breakfast competition.

Firstly, there's the chia seeds, which in simple words are a *superfood*, due to the fact that these tiny little black seeds are loaded with nutrients that support the brain and the body. The word *chia* is ancient Mayan and means strength.

The seeds are high in protein (so will keep you full), high in antioxidants (will slow down the aging process), as well as being high in omega-3, which will help to keep your heart healthy. And there is more—they are high in calcium, which helps keep our bones strong and helps prevent osteoporosis. And best of all, they're easy to prepare and can be eaten in so many ways.

Fresh figs are a tasty addition to this breakfast and supply a huge injection of antioxidants, with those anti-aging vitamins, which are A, E, and K, that can help also protect the body from disease.

Then let's not forget the apple, high in vitamin C, plus the high protein in the *fromage frais*, and then finally adding the cinnamon helps stimulate your metabolic rate, slightly increasing your calorie burn.

And limes are high in vitamin A and calcium, so give yourself an extra vitamin boost with this alongside your breakfast in the morning.

Great for skin, heart, weight loss and anti-aging.

Ingredients:

4 fresh figs

1 tablespoon chia seeds

1/4 pint unsweetened raspberry juice

1 tablespoon low-fat *fromage frais*

1 apple

Pinch of cinnamon

1 lime

Sparkling water

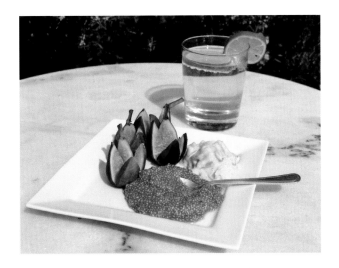

11

To make your chia-seed jam (you will not believe how simple this is), you need to allow the chia seeds to soak. I do mine overnight. Leave your chia seeds soaking in a glass topped up with your raspberry juice, and overnight they will absorb the juice and grow in size and soften in texture.

Cut and core your apple. Then chop it into tiny pieces and mix it in with your *fromage frais*. Add your sprinkle of cinnamon and mix thoroughly. Put your washed and sliced figs on a plate and add your apple and cheese mixture. Finally add your delicious chia-seed jam. Then wash it down with your fizzy lime.

This breakfast is rich in goodness, and you should feel full till lunchtime—oh yes, and feel fabulous.

Simple low-calorie hydrating zoodle salad

This little—well, actually big—salad of mine is super hydrating. You can whip this up in seconds, and its high water content means it keeps your body fully hydrated. Also, by being creative with your seasoning, you can make it absolutely mouth-watering. The benefits of this dish are that the key ingredients, courgette (also known as zucchini) and cucumber, are both high in vitamin K and C and dietary fibre, and the cucumber is over 90 per cent water, which keeps you fully hydrated and helps to eliminate toxins from your body.

Great for weight loss and skin.

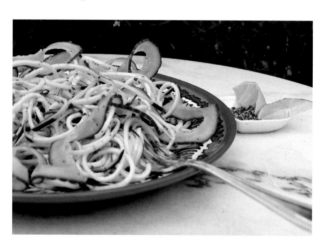

Ingredients:

1 courgette

1/4 cucumber

1 teaspoon olive oil

Seasoning

Slices of lemon and lime

I used a spiralizer to turn the courgette into what I refer to as *zoodles* (i.e., noodles out of zucchini), but if you don't have one, you can use a grater or a mandolin for the purpose. I also used this for the cucumber, but again you can just grate it. Drizzle some olive oil over this and also squeeze some fresh lemon and lime juice over it. Sprinkle on your seasoning. You can add cooked prawns or cooked chicken breast.

Chocolate-dipped apple wedges with crunchy strawberry pieces

My weakness is chocolate, and where there is a will, there is a way. This is one of my favourite ways to indulge guilt free. Using just one square of dark chocolate means I can sit back and enjoy this, and the good news is that dark chocolate is actually good for us! It can be good for improving blood flow, and it can help lower blood pressure. But this does not mean we should eat a bar a day! Melting it on to a piece of fruit means you only use a small amount, but it spreads on well so that you feel like you are eating much more than you are.

Great for boosting your immune system and heart health.

Ingredients:

1 square dark chocolate

1 apple

1 teaspoon dried strawberry pieces, or you can use dried raspberry if you prefer

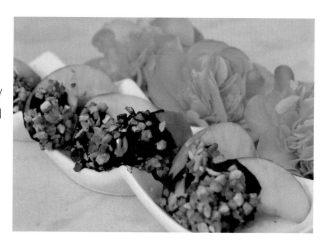

Wash, core and cut your apple into wedges. Melt 1 square of dark chocolate. Sprinkle some dried strawberry pieces (you can find these sold in most supermarkets) on to a flat plate.

Once the chocolate has melted, dip one end of your apple slice into it, and then sprinkle strawberry pieces on top. Place in the fridge to let it set.

Sexy salsa and salmon dinner

Okay, so this one I had to call a sexy dinner, as this is full of ingredients that have amazing effects on your appearance. This dish is high in omega-3s (the salmon), which is great for your skin; plus the good fats in the avocado help keep your skin plumped up, which helps reduce fine lines; and the delicious salsa has a secret ingredient, namely pomegranate. This will protect and strengthen skin cells on the surface and regenerate cells in the deeper layers of skin. So sit down in the early evening and enjoy this dinner, which is, let's face, it cheaper than going to the beauty salon for a facial, and it will get you better results, as we feed and treat our skin from the inside out.

Great for anti-aging and heart health.

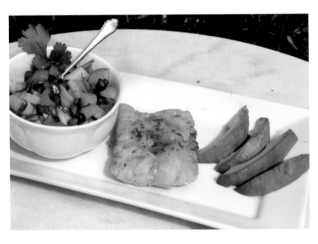

Ingredients:

1 salmon fillet

Bunch of coriander

1 apple

1 small avocado

1 small red onion

1/4 cucumber

Several cherry tomatoes

Handful of pomegranate seeds

First bake your salmon. Brush with a little olive oil, add some chopped chilli and coriander and cook for between 10-12 minutes at 220 °C (425 °F). Make sure your salmon is thoroughly cooked all the way through. Peel and slice your avocado.

For your salsa, finely chop the onion, cherry tomatoes, cucumber and apple. Then mix them together and pour a little balsamic vinegar over them. Then top with ripped coriander leaves and pomegranate seeds.

Avocado hummus

D for Delicious Dip. This is one of the best dips you can make, and again it's very easy. It contains pure ingredients, so you can dip away, knowing that you are eating clean food. You can have this with numerous vegetable crudités, such as cucumber sticks, carrot batons, celery stalks, florets of cauliflower and broccoli or, one of my favourites, red pepper. And red peppers are known to have a whole host of health benefits.

11

Great for heart health and energy levels.

Ingredients:

1 small tin of chickpeas

1 small avocado

1 teaspoon olive oil

1 lime

Cayenne pepper

Coarse black peppercorns

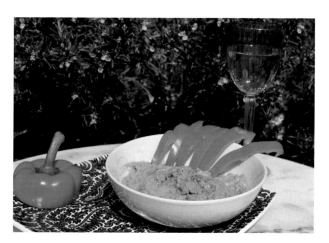

Heat the chickpeas in a pan. While they are cooking, peel your avocado and remove the stone. Then place it in a blender. Once the chickpeas are cooked, remove from heat and drain. Add to the blender. Squeeze in some lime juice and drizzle in a little oil. Then blend.

Place your dip in a bowl, and then drizzle a little oil on top and sprinkle on your seasoning. Serve with your favourite crunchy crudités.

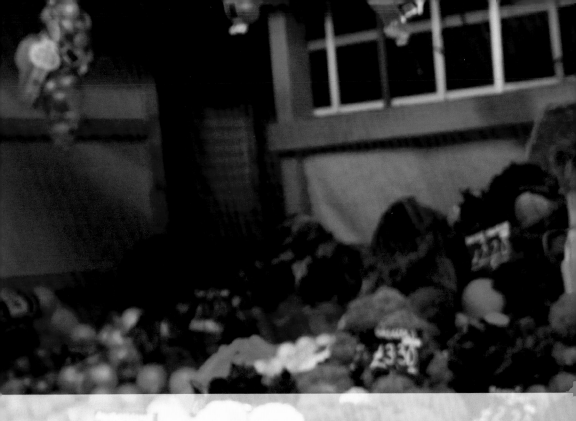

SHOPPING LIST

Make sure on your next shopping list you have just natural foods. And here is an example of a super healthy shopping list:

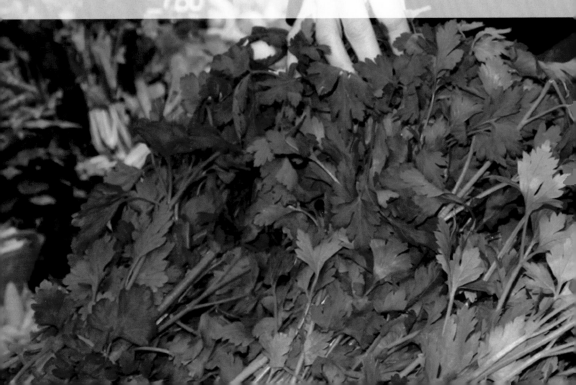

1 organic chicken
Salmon fillets
Tuna (in spring water)
Extra lean beef mince
Turkey mince
Fresh fish

Low-fat natural yoghurt
Cottage cheese
Eggs
Feta
Almonds
Walnuts
Spinach
Sweet potatoes
Courgettes
Onions
Cucumber
Tomatoes
Asparagus
Sugar snap peas
Sweetcorn
Red peppers
Chickpeas
Quinoa
Lentils

Brown rice
Sprouted seeds
Bananas
Frozen berries (great for smoothies)
Apples
Pears
Strawberries
Raisins
Pomegranates
Oat milk
Sparkling water

A good rule of thumb to use when it comes to preparing your foods is to stick with one of these methods of cooking: steaming, baking, poaching, grilling or stir-fry (using a very small amount of olive oil).

One of the best ways to give any dish or snack extra flavour is to use herbs and spices, so whether you pick fresh herbs from your garden—and nowadays you can buy some wonderful premade mini-herb gardens that grow on a window sill, so if you live in a flat you can still grow your own herbs—or buy some good spices—these are also stacked high in minerals so have major benefits as well as add lots of flavour—it is worth spending a little bit of money on some good-quality spices. Small markets are one of the best places you can get natural ingredients from a vast selection.

11

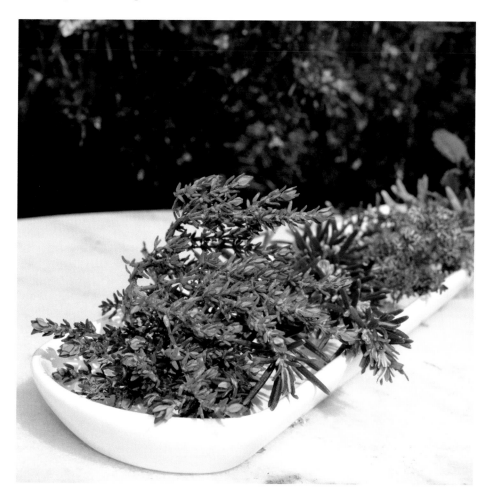

Some of the healthiest herbs and spices are:

sage,
rosemary,
turmeric,
chilli powder,
cinnamon,
ginger,
saffron and
parsley.

Make sure your diet is full of delicious clean foods.

As you can see healthy clean foods can be vibrant, delicious and simple to eat, so keep it simple, and you will look and feel your best.

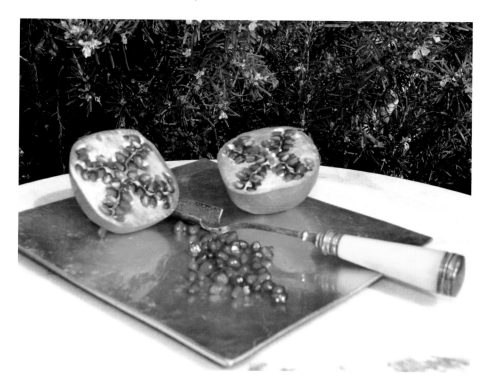

12 MOTIVATION

To me this is one of the most important parts of any fitness and nutrition plan, as our mind is the boss of our body and has the power to either make us want to jump up and put on our trainers or stay on the sofa and eat the wrong foods. We need to know how we can convince our mind to overcome those hurdles which we all have every now and again.

EXCUSES BUSTED

To start with, this section has the most common reasons that we say no and think that we can't do things, so if you find one day you're thinking of turning to one of these excuses to not to exercise, then read my solution.

Excuse 1: I have not got time today.

My solution: What about just 5 minutes? I am convinced that you have 5 minutes, which is just 300 seconds! Just remember that your goals are worth finding the time for. You could just do one round of your toning workouts, or just set a timer and do as much as you can in that time.

Excuse 2: I am too tired.

My solution: Okay, with this second most common excuse comes some irony, because if you are tired, then sitting down will, believe it or not, just make you feel more tired, so you need to switch on that determination button and just start working out. You will instantly feel energized, and instead of feeling tired you will feel alive. Think of exercise as your phone's battery charger. When your phone's battery is running out, you then charge it up, and it has a new lease of life. Well this is what will happen to you the minute you put on those trainers and do my workouts. So combat this excuse by making yourself do the workout, as that in itself is the cure to feeling tired.

Excuse 3: My children are on school holidays, so I won't be able to train.

My solution: Well it's great that they are around, because you can be a great role model to them when they see mummy being fit. Get them to do all the counting for the exercise, and then go with them for a walk. Get them to take part. Obviously don't get them doing your exercises, but you could get them to do some fun star jumps or other kids' activities alongside yours.

Excuse 4: I feel too fat and heavy and find exercise uncomfortable.

My solution: First, find some comfy clothes to work out in, and even if, say, for just two weeks you simply do a 10-minute walk around the block, this will reduce your body fat, and you will soon find exercise feels easier and your body moves more freely.

Excuse 5: It is too cold to exercise!

My solution: Top tip of mine here: Leave your workout clothes on a radiator. If you are a morning girl, you can jump out of bed and get warm in your workout gear, or you can have them waiting nice and toasty when you get back from work, ready for you to jump into and start working out.

So the only time for you to say no to exercise is if you are unwell or have an injury. And remember, you don't have to do it every day of the week—just four to five times. So we really can find the time and motivation. And it is so worth the investment of your time and effort, as you will feel GREAT afterwards.

Fitness motivation mantras

If you need some extra motivation, here are some of the best mantras, and if one really jumps out at you, take a photo of it and have it on your phone and computer as a contact prompt. You will also find lots more on my Pinterest boards at

www.Pinterest.com/lwrfitness/

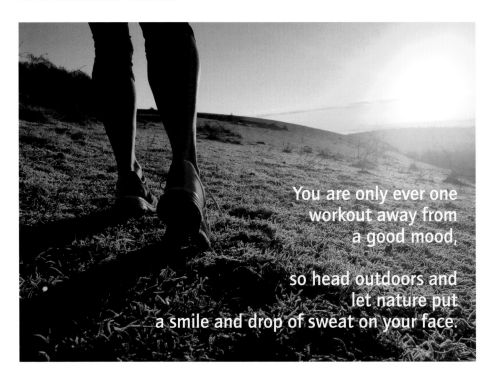

12

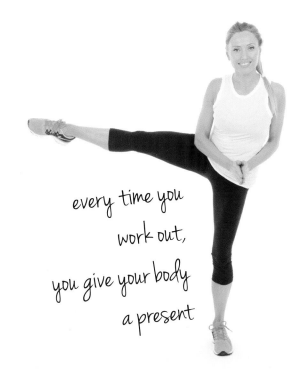

every time you
work out,
you give your body
a present

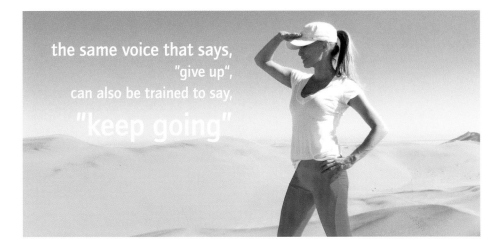

the same voice that says,
"give up",
can also be trained to say,
"keep going"

13 READYMADE WORKOUTS

In this section of the book, I have carefully selected the ideal workouts for you for each specific routine. Again this will combine toning and a mix of cardio and will be a 21-day plan.

BRIDAL BOOT CAMP WORKOUT

This is all about toning those areas that are on show on your big wedding day. This workout looks at improving your upper-body posture and sculpting beautiful shoulders and sleek-toned arms so that you can feel confident all day in your dress. We also work on toning deep into those waist muscles so that you can have that beautiful feminine shape on your wedding day. For the cardio workout we are going to follow the powerwalking plan, as this will help strip any excess body fat and help keep your muscles super toned.

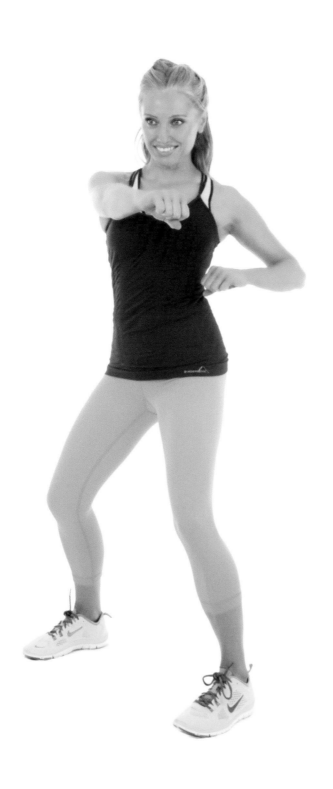

The workout

Exercise 1: Curtsey (page 69)

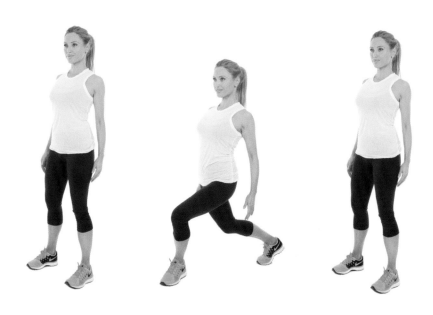

Beginner: 12-16 reps, 2 sets
Intermediate: 18-22 reps, 2 sets
Advanced: 20 reps, 3 sets

Exercise 2: Sexy Shoulder Sculptor (page 115)

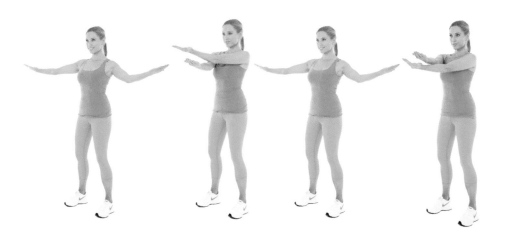

Beginner: 20 reps, 3 sets

Intermediate: 30 reps, 3 sets

Advanced: 50 reps, 3 sets

Exercise 3: Spreading Wings Lift (page 133)

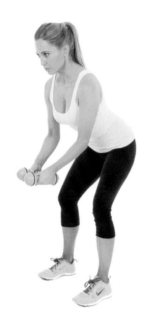 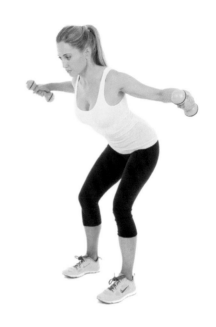

Beginner: 10-12 reps, 2 sets

Intermediate: 12-14 reps, 3 sets

Advanced: 20 reps, 3 sets

Exercise 4: Wonder Bust Press (page 98)

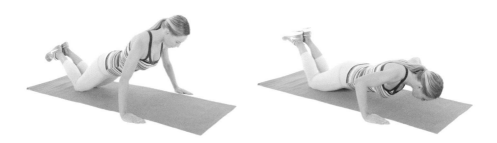

Beginner: 6-8 reps, 2 sets

Intermediate: 10-12 reps, 2 sets

Advanced: 20 reps, 2 sets

Exercise 5: Facedown Ab Crunch (page 46)

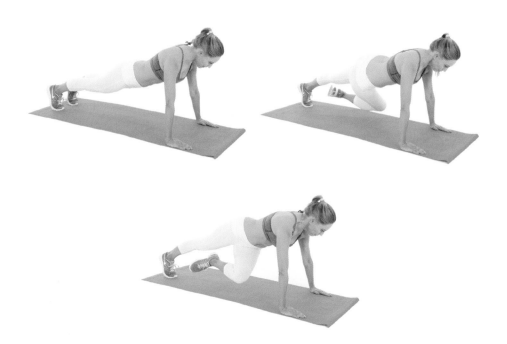

Beginner: 14-18 reps, 2 sets
Intermediate: 8-20 reps, 3 sets
Advanced: 30 reps, 4 sets

The 21-day plan

13

Bridal boot camp workout		
	Week 1	Week 2	Week 3
Monday	**Bridal boot camp workout**	16-Minute Fat-Burning Powerwalk	16-Minute Fat-Burning Powerwalk and **Bridal boot camp workout**
Tuesday	16-Minute Fat-Burning Powerwalk	**Bridal boot camp workout**	**Bridal boot camp workout**
Wednesday	**Bridal boot camp workout**	Rest	16-Minute Fat-Burning Powerwalk
Thursday	Rest	16-Minute Fat-Burning Powerwalk	**Bridal boot camp workout**
Friday	16-Minute Fat-Burning Powerwalk	**Bridal boot camp workout**	Rest
Saturday	**Bridal boot camp workout**	16-Minute Fat-Burning Powerwalk	**Bridal boot camp workout**
Sunday	16-Minute Fat-Burning Powerwalk	**Bridal boot camp workout**	16-Minute Fat-Burning Powerwalk

SOS BIKINI WORKOUT

If you have a holiday looming up fast and want to swap your old swimsuit for a bikini, then stick to this 21-day plan, and you can lounge by the pool feeling fabulous in your bikini. For this workout I am giving you two cardio sessions: the powerwalk and the step workout, as the walk will help burn off excess body fat and the step workout is going to give you that perfect butt and slender thighs for your bikini.

The workout

Exercise 1: Brazilian Butt Squat Drop (page 66)

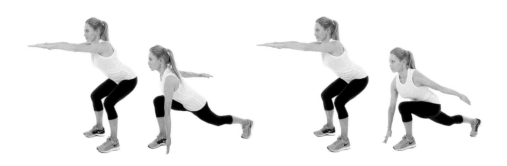

Beginner: 6-8 reps, 2 sets
Intermediate: 10-12 reps, 3 sets
Advanced: 16-20 reps, 4 sets

Exercise 2: Book Press (page 102)

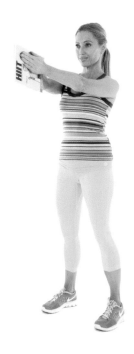

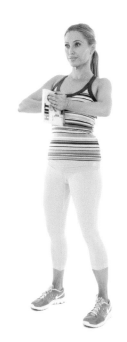

Beginner:	12-14 reps, 2 sets
Intermediate:	14-18 reps, 3 sets
Advanced:	20-25 reps, 4 sets

Exercise 3: Ballerina's Butt (page 68)

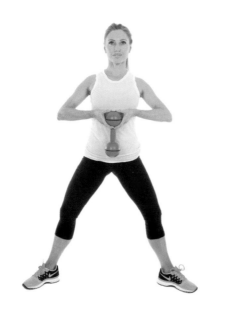
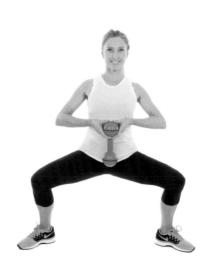

Beginner: 12-14 reps, 2 sets
Intermediate: 16-20 reps, 3 sets
Advanced: 30 reps, 4 sets

Exercise 4: Ab Makeover (page 47)

13

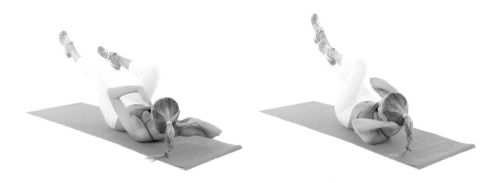

Beginner: 12-14 reps, 2 sets
Intermediate: 18-20 reps, 3 sets
Advanced: 30 reps, 4 sets

Exercise 5: Two-Step Lean Legs Lift (page 84)

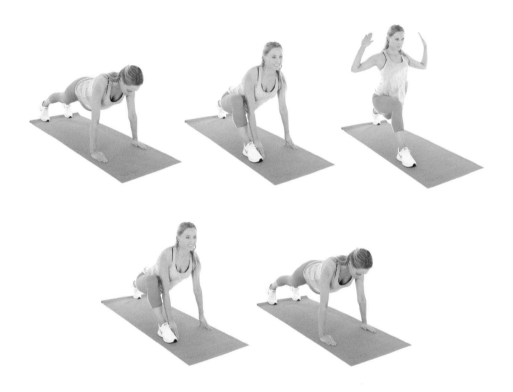

Beginner:	4 reps, 2 sets
Intermediate:	8 reps, 3 sets
Advanced:	12 reps, 4 sets

13.2.2 The 21-day plan

SOS bikini workout		
	Week 1	**Week 2**	**Week 3**
Monday	SOS Bikini workouts	16-Minute Fat-Burning Powerwalk	SOS Bikini workouts
Tuesday	16-Minute Fat-Burning Powerwalk	Rest	10 Steps to Perfect Tone Workout
Wednesday	10 Steps to Perfect Tone Workout	SOS Bikini workouts	16-Minute Fat-Burning Powerwalk
Thursday	SOS Bikini workouts	10 Steps to Perfect Tone Workout	SOS Bikini workouts
Friday	16-Minute Fat-Burning Powerwalk	SOS Bikini workouts	Rest
Saturday	SOS Bikini workouts	16-Minute Fat-Burning Powerwalk	SOS Bikini workouts
Sunday	Rest	SOS Bikini workouts	16-Minute Fat-Burning Powerwalk

LOOK 10 YEARS YOUNGER WORKOUT

By eating the right foods and doing the right exercise we can all turn back the body clock and look younger, healthier and feel fitter, without having to go under the knife or spend a small fortune on expensive lotions and potions. Our body has a hormone known as the *human growth hormone* (HGH), and this is the hormone that keeps us looking youthful. After the age of 30 or even a little earlier the body slows down the production of this hormone, and that is why our skin may not be a plump—HGH is responsible for helping keep our collagen fully plumped up. The good news is exercise helps stimulate this hormone, increasing its natural daily production. So the *beauty* of exercise is that it really can help you look younger, stay in shape and keep off the middle-age spread. For this workout I have picked exercises that work big muscle groups to really help with full HGH stimulation, and these moves also help lift certain areas that can sag. We will tone and tighten them back up.

For your cardio you can chose between the powerwalking workout on page 148 or the running workout on page 151, as both of these will yield great results. Simply choose the one you enjoy the most. I really recommend you try some of my tasty recipes from the food section as these are all loaded with lots of antioxidants which are great for the condition of our skin, keeping it looking more radiant and keeping our hair shiny and nails strong.

The workout

Exercise 1: Towel Squeeze (page 103)

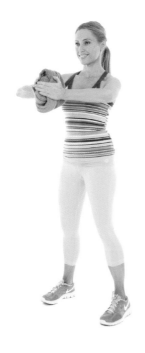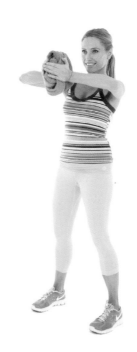

Beginner: 12 reps, 2 sets
Intermediate: 16 reps, 3 sets
Advanced: 20 reps, 4 sets

Exercise 2: Banish Bingo Wing Squeeze (page 114)

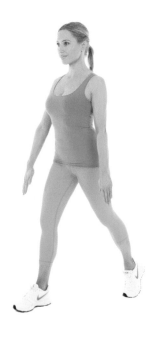 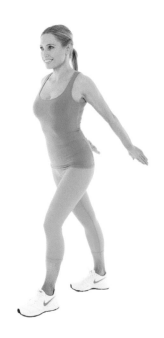

Beginner: 50 reps, 1 sets
Intermediate: 50 reps, 2 sets
Advanced: 100 reps, 2 sets

Exercise 3: Love Your Legs Lunge (page 79)

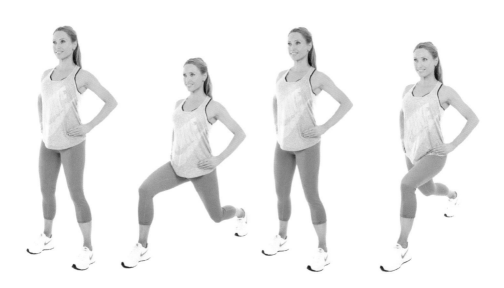

Beginner: 10-12 reps, 2 sets

Intermediate: 14-18 reps, 3 sets

Advanced: 30 reps, 4 sets

Exercise 4: Superwoman (page 136)

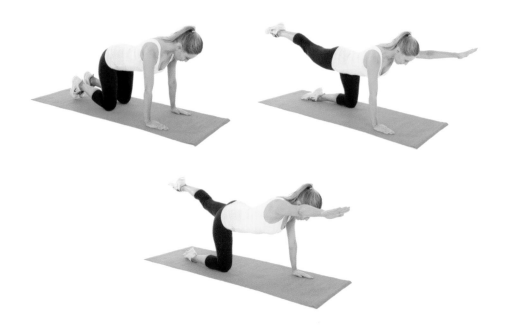

Beginner: 8 reps, 2 sets
Intermediate: 10 reps, 3 sets
Advanced: 20 reps, 3 sets

Exercise 5: Squat (page 65)

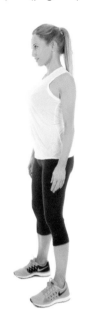 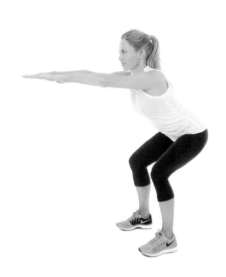

Beginner: 12-14 reps, 2 sets
Intermediate: 20-26 reps, 3 sets
Advanced: 30 reps, 4 sets

Exercise 6: Waist Inch Loss Twist (page 51)

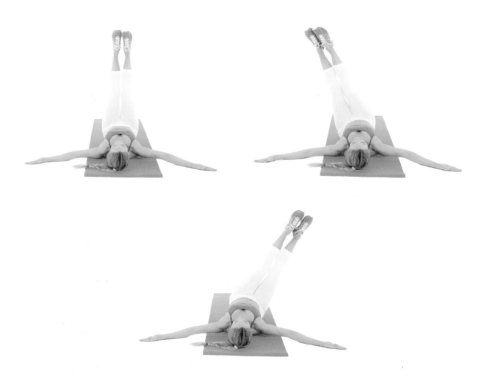

Beginner: 6-8 reps, 2 sets

Intermediate: 12-14 reps, 3 sets

Advanced: 16-20 reps, 4 sets

The 21-day plan

Look 10 years younger workout			
	Week 1	Week 2	Week 3
Monday	Look 10 years younger workout	Walk or run	Look 10 years younger workout
Tuesday	Walk or run	Look 10 years younger workout	Rest
Wednesday	Walk or run	Look 10 years younger workout	Walk or run
Thursday	Look 10 years younger workout	Rest	Look 10 years younger workout
Friday	Walk or run	Look 10 years younger workout	Walk or run
Saturday	Look 10 years younger workout	Walk or run	Look 10 years younger workout
Sunday	Rest	Look 10 years younger workout	Walk or run

4-MINUTE QUICK WORKOUT

This workout is designed for when you only have a few minutes but want to burn off fat. It's all you need to do. To complete the 4-Minute Quick Workout, do 20 seconds of the Inner and Outer Thigh Sculpting Jump; then have a 10-second rest period in which you march on the spot; repeat this and keep doing it for a total of 4 minutes, which is 8 rounds of each. The benefit of this is it works your lower body, and these intervals of 20 seconds help torch calories fast. This can increase the amount of calories your body burns all day. Always warm up and stretch first, and cool down properly at the end.

Exercise 1: Inner and Outer Thigh Sculpting Jump

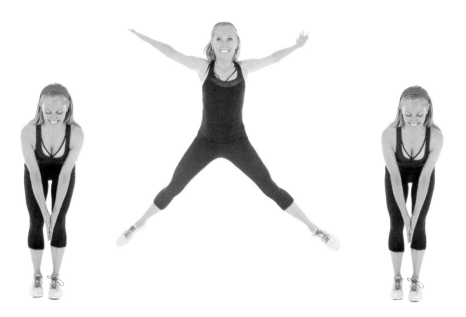

Starting in a deep squat position, hold then jump up as high as you can, trying to get your arms and legs out wide. Land softly back in your deep squat position. Repeat for exactly 20 seconds. Then go straight into exercise 2.

Exercise 2: March on the Spot

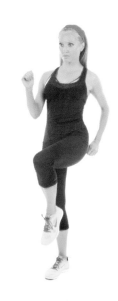

March on the spot for 10 seconds. This is your recovery time, so you don't need to march fast. Just keep your body moving and take in some nice, deep breaths.

Repeat both exercises for a total of 4 minutes. Follow this exact workout in realtime with me on my YouTube Channel, this video is called "Hiit Workout—4 Minutes Fat Burning"

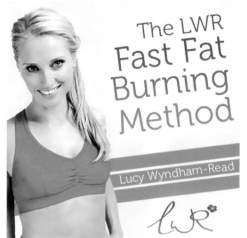

This workout is available as an audio download on Amazon and iTunes in which I coach you through the full workout.

ACKNOWLEDGMENTS

Firstly my family, as they have always encouraged me and supported me on this great journey; they have been there for me every single step of the way. I owe everything to them all. And special individual thanks to Mum, Dad, Uncle Keith for all his hard work with proofreading and editing, Aunt Mandy, Jess and Johnny, and my scrumptious nieces Hatty, Mimi and Princess Lucy, and my wonderful nephew Tom.

A big thank you to Michael, who has sacrificed plenty of early mornings to head out for outdoor photo opportunities, for his ongoing support and belief. And to Tony Stevens for his great photography. You all have been part of this book and my journey.

Then lastly I would like to dedicate this book to my fiancé Mike, who was sadly killed many years ago but who has always remained my shining star. True love never dies.

Come and say hi to me on my social media and let me know how you have got on with all your workouts:

 LWRFitness Channel

 @lucywyndhamread

 @lucywyndhamread

 LWR Fitness

 LWR Fitness

ONE FINAL NOTE

Never doubt yourself, and never give up. This book is now your tool to keep you on the healthy road, giving you a lifestyle that is full of energy and well-being. Lucy x

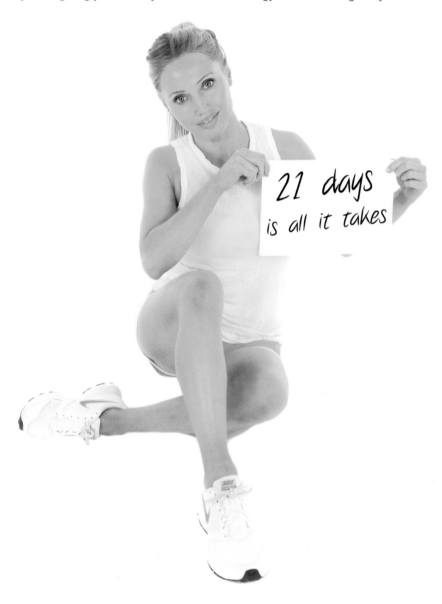